# Breathing for Life: Our Stories

# Breathing for Life: Our Stories

## *As We Breathe, We Hope*

People affected by Pulmonary
Disease who were willing to share
their stories

authorHOUSE®

*AuthorHouse™*
*1663 Liberty Drive*
*Bloomington, IN 47403*
*www.authorhouse.com*
*Phone: 1-800-839-8640*

*Published by AuthorHouse    2/27/2012*

*ISBN: 978-1-4670-3136-3 (sc)*
*ISBN: 978-1-4670-3135-6 (ebk)*

*Editors,  Dr. Cynthia L.Marshall and Dan W. Coleman*

# CONTENTS

## EN ROUTE TO A TRANSPLANT . . . DESTINATION REACHED 11/11/11

## SOME BATTLES ARE WON ON THE OTHER SIDE

*This book is dedicated to all of the individuals who have been diagnosed with a lung disease, those previously diagnosed and passed through this life and those of us still surviving and those who may one day have to hear a doctor's diagnosis of lung disease. To all of the friends and family members whose lives have been affected personally and to all of the groups, which labor so diligently to elevate awareness, raise and distribute funds to continue research and find cures to help all of us breathe a better life, we say thank you.*

*I would also like to dedicate this volume to all of the wonderful and marvelous staff at the Duke Center for Living Fitness Center (Pulmonary Rehab Program) for your support.*

*Personally, I have to thank my God for giving me the health, wellness, knowledge and strength to realize this project from start to finish.*

# Acknowledgments

I am most grateful to my editors. Dr. Cynthia L. Marshall and Dan W. Coleman. To my proof reader, Kathy Kling who so graciously volunteered for the position. A special indebtedness to Joanne Schum, author of *Taking Flight: Inspirational Stories of Lung Transplantation,* for your precious time devoted to me as I navigated through this unfamiliar territory.

I recall one very frustrating day when my friend, Rita Price, inspired me to and beyond the point of no retreat with the words, "God always wants us to do things that give others hope". Thanks also to her daughters, Charity and Hope, for allowing me so much of their mother's attention during this project.

To Tyler Garrett, whose support and belief in me pushed me through many ruts, and also for keeping my technology problems under control. I could not have asked for a better son.

Credit goes to my inspiration and motivation for life, and in life—my granddaughter, Taysia, to you, darling one, I say thank you for being so inspired by granny's project. I love you.

To those that helped me stay encouraged and committed to the end. To God for placing people in my life right when I needed them most, I am forever grateful.

Countless and abundant thanks to the fund-raising crew, individual financial contributors and to the courageous conquerors of pulmonary disease who were willing to share their stories.

*Sometimes we take for granted the air that we breathe until we are faced with lung disease . . .*

# Foreword

Lung disease affects every breath you take. Patients with lung disease know this well and experience discomfort with breathing 24 hours a day. The most common form of lung disease is called Chronic Obstructive Pulmonary Disease (COPD), a condition that encompasses chronic bronchitis and emphysema. With COPD, the airways become narrow and the lungs fail to empty properly. COPD is estimated to affect as many as 20 million Americans and is now the fourth leading cause of death in the United States. Asthma, another airway disease also affects millions of patients but, unlike COPD, there is significant reversibility of the airway narrowing. Less common forms of lung disease include tissue inflammation that causes scarring in the lung (fibrosis), blood vessel abnormalities (pulmonary hypertension and vasculitis) and lung cancer. Taken together, this family of diseases significantly limits the lifestyle of tens of millions of patients, costs the healthcare system billions of dollars, and ultimately can cut short productive lives.

Over the last two decades, significant advances have been made in the management of a variety of lung diseases. For example, in COPD new classes of bronchodilators and anti-inflammatory medications have made living with COPD much easier. Supplemental oxygen in the right COPD patients can also dramatically improve function and lung volume reduction surgery can significantly lengthen life in COPD patients with specific types of emphysema. In asthma, there have also been advances in new bronchodilator and anti-inflammatory therapies that have made living with this disease much more tolerable. In other forms of lung disease, clinical trials are ongoing to find better ways of managing them. This is particularly true in the blood vessel diseases and in lung cancer. Perhaps, however, the most important recent advancement in the management of end stage lung disease has been the improvement in lung transplantation. One year survival rates from lung transplantation are now greater than 90% and longer, more productive lives are being experienced by lung transplant recipients.

Along with all of these medical developments has been a growing awareness of the importance of the power of patient attitude and involvement in disease management. When patients understand their disease better they know better how to work with the healthcare team to maximize function, optimize long term care plans, and deal with exacerbations of their disease. This involvement often involves supervised exercise through rehabilitation programs. The evidence is overwhelming that participating in formal rehabilitation programs greatly enhances functional status and quality of life. These programs also help patients understand better how to prevent the complications of their disease. In short, integrating principles of rehabilitation with optimal medical management is allowing patients to live life to the fullest despite these chronic illnesses.

This book is dedicated to those patients who have embraced this concept. This book tells of the struggles and the successes in a variety of different clinical situations. These stories are truly inspirational to those of us in the healthcare profession and should serve as an inspiration to all those who deal with chronic lung disease, both the patients and the caregivers. Life with chronic lung disease does not have to be a debilitating end to an active and productive life. There is hope and these stories are testimonies to that hope.

Neil R. MacIntyre, MD

# Disclaimer

Stories shared in this book are personal, told by people who know first-hand what it means to live with lung disease. The stories are recounted in each author's own words, reflecting each author's unique perspective, including their religious beliefs. These stories are for informational purposes only. They are not intended to be nor should they be taken as medical opinions, evaluations, advice, or treatment suggestion. If you, or someone you know, are/is experiencing pulmonary difficulties, you should schedule a medical consult with a certified health care provider who can perform a medical evaluation and diagnosis of your condition. Always consult your doctor before making any decision affecting your health.

Please be advised that, although every effort has been made to ensure the correct usage of grammar and punctuation, we nevertheless defer to our original intent which is to preserve the original voice of each writer. The views expressed in these accounts, including any factual errors, omissions, or misstatements, are the sole responsibility of the respective authors. The publisher assumes no responsibility for any statements or assertions made by any of the authors.

While many of the authors have received care through the Duke University Medical System, this publication is in no way affiliated with, endorsed by or produced in conjunction with Duke University.

All rights are reserved by the authors of the book. No part of this book may be copied or otherwise reproduced without the expressed written permission of the authors. The authors reserve the rights to alter, amend, or change information.

# AS WE BREATHE, WE HOPE

# My Lungs and Me

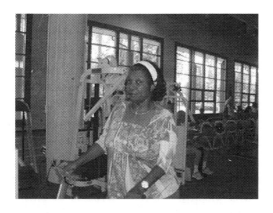

## *A Story of Living With Bronchiectasis*

My name is Catherine Lee Brockington. I was twice married and twice divorced.

Being on oxygen since 2008 has really changed my life. When I was a child, my mother told me I was born with a spot on my lungs the size of a quarter and that I died twice on the table at Duke Hospital. As a child I was not getting treatment and care as I do now. My parents did the best they could with little knowledge about the disease. I had a very hard time. I was not introduced to an inhaler until I was grown and away from my parents. I don't recall having one when I was growing up at home. I do remember walking backwards in the cold weather and on windy days. You know God was taking care of me. GOD I THANK YOU.

I moved to Seattle, Washington, at the age of nineteen with my first husband who, then, was in the Army. I was a lean, mean and a good looking machine until I started having babies. My asthma stayed under control. I even smoked back then. I stayed busy running behind four kids; two in pampers and two driving me to drink (diet coke). Imagine that! In different climates my asthma can be good or bad. Living out in Seattle, Washington, was good for me until Mount Saint Helen erupted. The beaches are good for my asthma also. Let the truth be told; I didn't start having breathing problems or coughing until I quit smoking and I only smoked four a day. It is what it is. I'm blessed and God knows best.

I started having problems, or should I say my asthma has gotten worse, over the last 10 to 15 years. I was referred to Raleigh Pulmonary and Allergy Consultants years ago under the care of Dr. Kunstling, a great doctor. I was treated with pills, inhalers, and more pills, but I still did not get any better. I started the monthly injections of XOLAIR® for asthma until I researched the injection and found out it can cause cancer. I told Dr. Kunstling I was stopping the shot and why. A couple of weeks later, I was asked if I would like to participate in a trial study on XOLAIR® for patients who were stopping the injection. The research was done at Duke Asthma Allergy and Airway Clinic. They would watch me for five years to see if I get cancer since I stopped the injection. *Lord, I come to you as humbly as I know how asking that you forgive me of all of my short comings and sins. Please father keep me cancer free Amen.*

The good thing that has happened to me since I stopped taking the Xolair® injection and started my clinical trial is that I met the greatest doctor at Duke Asthma Allergy and Airway Center. I was in one of the exam rooms waiting on Denise, another great lady at Duke, to start the trial procedures. I started coughing, and coughing and more coughing. Dr. Lugogo came in and asked me if she could be my doctor and help me with that cough. I immediately said yes.

The next day my records were transferred from Raleigh Pulmonary and Allergy Consultants to Duke Asthma, Allergy and Airway Clinic. I knew I had a lung disease along with asthma, remembering the spot on my lung. I thought the spot had come back. However, I didn't know what type. Dr. Lugogo explained it all to me. She sent me for blood work, a chest x-ray, a CAT scan, and an ultrasound. Dr. Lugogo diagnosed me with bronchiectasis, a fungus of the lungs that if caught at an early stage, can be treated. Unfortunately, I was diagnosed in 2003 but was never treated or told that I had the disease. I did research and found my old medical records and found my early diagnoses. I remembered Dr. Lugogo telling me if the disease were caught at an early stage it would be treatable.

Dr. Lugogo explained to me that my disease was incurable due to years going untreated. Imagine that! She explained that I must stay up on my medicines and exercise to lose weight to one day go for a transplant; I would need to drop to about 130 to 140 pounds.

I think the biggest mistake I made was getting too dependent on oxygen. When Rex Hospital sent me home with oxygen, I wish I would have just used it when needed. Now, I am hooked just like I was when I smoked. Dr. Lugogo had mentioned to me several times that she was going to wean me off of oxygen. Only time will tell.

*However; as long as I keep my faith in God I know everything will work out. These are all our trials and tribulation. It is up to us to stand the test of times. God has given my doctor the knowledge; I will listen and obey. I still need the Big Foot Prints to continue to walk with me day and night and hold me tight in his arms.*

I would be lying if I said I have good days all the time. I get very upset at times and cry and hate everybody. I get tired of moving slowly, breathing deeply and wearing the nasal cannula, carrying the oxygen, and not being able to do the things I used to do are hard. I would get mad at my parents for not doing follow up maintenance. I was one unhappy person. My second husband didn't understand my needs, or my strength even. Two people loving each other but didn't know how to love.

I hope one day . . . wrong word . . . I KNOW I will get better one day because of the wonderful people at Duke Center for

Living: Rebecca Crouch, Carol Carson, Sheila Shearer, David Best, Sara Johnson, Courtney Frankel, Sarah Peterson, Wanda, Rebecca 2, last but not least, Dr. Macintyre, are all great physical therapists and doctor who work real hard to get their patients moving and not giving up. I am a witness. Thank God they believed in me when I didn't believe in myself. One time I lost 15 lbs. I was very happy for myself. I loved hearing Sara tell me "Catherine you are looking good". It's words like that that keep you going. Rebecca and Carol would push and tell me the importance of exercise, walking and biking. I got sick back to back, in and out the hospital, a week at a time. My immune system is very low, and I can catch a cold from someone easily. I enjoy coming to the center. I'm not alone in this lung battle. I have nice people to whom to talk I can laugh. I can cry. I have learned so much from the different classes taught by the therapists. To them all, I say, "Thank you."

I will try not to get mad anymore about my lung disease; it is what it is.

*As long as I continue to seek the Kingdom I'll be all right. My God will keep me and guide me.*

To end my story is not to end at all because I'm not done yet. Whatever God has in store for me I will accept because he knows my heart, which is to get better. Did I tell you I sing in the Senior Choir at New Bethel Missionary Baptist Church on the 1st Sunday? Come visit sometime. Every once in a while I lead a song. Continue to keep me in your prayers and likewise I will keep you in my prayers.

Beverly, thank you for giving me a chance to tell some of my story. I didn't write using the fancy words because it would have been all fake. This is Catherine Elaine Lee/Brockington and this is my story. To be continued . . .

*Catherine E. Lee/Brockington*

# Living with Atypical Idiopathic Pulmonary Fibrosis

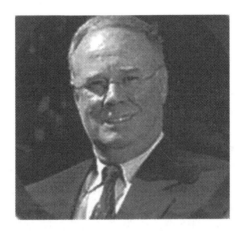

*A Story of "Never, Never Give Up!"*

I am a retired 67-years-old high technology company executive and business owner who has lived and worked in the Research Triangle Park area of North Carolina for over 30 years. Before that, I was in the U.S. Army and worked for Bell Telephone Laboratories. For the better part of the past three years, I have been living with the knowledge that I have a lung disease with an unknown prognosis closely akin to idiopathic pulmonary fibrosis (IPF). Though it is little known outside of the pulmonary medicine community, IPF is 100% fatal without a lung transplant, killing 40,000 people each year, approximately the same number who die from breast cancer.

The survival rate for IPF is only one percent and these are people who are fortunate enough to receive a lung transplant. In the late fall of 2007, I was diagnosed with IPF after experiencing several months of unexplained coughing and increasing shortness of breath. My doctor was a pulmonologist in nearby Raleigh. Following his preliminary diagnosis, this private practice pulmonologist referred me to a research pulmonologist at UNC Hospitals where the IPF diagnosis was confirmed. The UNC pulmonologist, a well-known lung cancer specialist, suggested that I see an IPF specialist. She highly recommended Dr. Paul Noble, one of the leading IPF experts in the world. Dr. Noble, who had recently moved from Yale to head the Pulmonary Division at Duke University Medical Center, responded immediately and scheduled an appointment to see me in his clinic.

Dr. Noble thought the diagnosis of IPF was likely but some atypical features identified on the high resolution chest CAT Scan raised the possibility that my disease was not typical IPF. I was started on aggressive immunosuppressive therapy. Most vivid in my memory on my first visit was his explanation to me that I have an extremely serious lung disease, and that, " . . . people with IPF in an accelerated phase can at times expect to live their lives in months, not years." This statement obviously got my attention!

I very much appreciated Dr. Noble's frankness as well as his serious and thoughtful plan to help me attempt to beat the odds through medication and pulmonary rehabilitation. His forthrightness enabled me to start planning for all eventualities during the life I had remaining and to put priorities in place that are consistent with my personal and family values.

I determined that my top priority must be to survive. Otherwise, I could not accomplish anything else. I had to think of my family members and be in a reasonable quality of life to enjoy them. Having a dedicated wife of 46 years, two fine, grown sons and daughters-in-law, plus six wonderful grandchildren, all of whom I deeply care about, motivated me to do everything within my control to survive. With survival and a decent quality of life at the top of my priority list, I next turned to what would be my legacy should I succumb to this dreaded disease. With my sons well-established in their businesses and their families happy and growing, my thoughts turned to my six grandchildren. Obviously, I very much desired that they would become my greatest legacy. So, I began to spend as much time as possible with all six of them—the oldest a beautiful nine-years-old girl plus five younger boys ranging from ages eight down to three years. I passed on family stories and enjoyed what we could do together, including playing Wii and other games at home, going to the beach and lakes swimming, fishing, and science projects. My desire has been to provide enrichment opportunities and assist their parents in preparing these young people for happy and successful lives.

In our family, love and service to others has been my wife's wonderfully articulated mantra for the entire time we have been married. Our boys fully understand and practice this approach to life and I want my grandchildren to do so also.
Never one to exercise regularly since I was in the Army, priority one, survival, led me to fully commit to the Pulmonary Rehab Program at the Duke Center for Living (CFL). This world-renowned program is led by Dr. Rebecca Crouch. Participation in this exercise-intensive program is required for all Duke pulmonary patients seeking a lung transplant. Following graduation from this 23 day program, I joined the on-going Pulmonary Rehab Graduate Program.

After participating in the Graduate Program at the CFL for a few months, I began to experience a further improvement in my ability to breathe, and, very importantly, in my pulmonary function numbers during exercise. The more aggressively I exercised, the less I depended upon supplemental oxygen. One day, after notifying the Pulmonary Rehab staff, I began to carefully exercise without oxygen. Miraculously, as confirmed by periodically observing my pulse throughout the exercise, my blood oxygen stayed well above the minimum saturation levels. I found that I could perform the prescribed floor exercises, arms and legs strength training, and aggressive cardiovascular exercise without the three liters per minute of oxygen.

During this time, I also successfully underwent a very extensive qualifying physical examination prescribed by the

Duke Lung Transplant team. I am sure the doctors were puzzled when my pulmonary function numbers began increasing instead of decreasing, an uncommon occurrence with typical IPF. They began, too, to question my IPF diagnosis. More data would become available when I later underwent a true lung biopsy.

Viewing a possible lung transplant as a safety net, I continue to visit the Duke Center for Living five days a week where I exercise for approximately two hours each visit. I lost weight and became physically stronger. As confirmed by periodic pulmonary function and 6 minute walk tests at the Duke Pulmonary clinic, my lung function was consistently above acceptable levels. I was able to both play with my grandchildren inside and outside and enjoy traveling to such places as the Canadian Rockies and the coast of Maine with my wife.

Unfortunately, this process has not been without interruption. Responding to moderate-to-severe reflux disease discovered during the extensive physical examination, I underwent a "stomach wrap" (Nissan fundoplication), a minimally invasive operation whose goal is to reduce the impact of reflux disease on lungs. Although I have not had a lung transplant, reflux disease, or G.E.R.D., is thought by some pulmonologists to be damaging to both old lungs and new.

The next interruption occurred when I developed an unexplained additional cough, and my pulmonary function numbers began to drop. Dr. Noble recommended I undergo a real lung biopsy in order to get further insight into what was going on inside my lungs. The Duke surgeon did a great job with the lung biopsy. I very soon returned to my exercise routine at the Center for Living. The lung biopsy showed that I have a form of Non-Specific Interstitial Pneumonia (NSIP) in addition to atypical IPF. In response, Dr. Noble prescribed an increased amount of prednisone. My pulmonary function numbers returned to their previous readings after a couple of months, resulting in the prednisone dose gradually being reduced.

I was not so fortunate with the next interruption in my pulmonary rehab regimen. During the Thanksgiving holidays last year, I acquired RSV, a very serious pulmonary virus that is most often seen in infants. With my weakened lungs and immune system and a sharply higher fever, a late evening visit to the Duke Medical Center emergency room became necessary. Uncontrolled coughing to the point of being physically painful characterized my hospital stay. During this time, led by Dr. Noble and the lung transplant team, the entire Duke pulmonary community, as well as the staff of the hospital, wrapped its collective arms around me to discover what was wrong and identify fixes. Following confirmation of RSV, I was sent home since there is no known treatment for this virus.

Unfortunately, my pulmonary function numbers had gone down, possibly as a result of the RSV. Fortunately, after a couple of weeks at home I recovered sufficiently to return to my pulmonary rehab program at the Center for Living. The good news is that I have been able to continue with my pulmonary rehab program, feeling stronger each day while my pulmonary function numbers remain acceptable.

In addition to highly valued time with my grandchildren and my Church, where I know many prayers are heard and answered, several hobbies help keep me interested in living. These hobbies include writing my second book rigorously documenting with primary sources a Civil War regiment from South Carolina, repairing and restoring vintage 1920's radios, and enjoying Amateur Radio. Church and my faith continue to be very important to me as are my social friends and colleagues from many years in business.

In summary, for nearly three years I have been an exception to what most frequently happens to patients with IPF, reaffirming that my IPF is atypical. During this time, I have, for the most part, enjoyed a high quality of life. I have become convinced that exercising to the limits of my blood oxygen saturation level can be important in delaying the need for a lung transplant. The caring staff and dedicated patients at the Duke Center for Living have become my new friends. During the nearly three years I have been at the Center, I have seen many pulmonary patients begin the program slowly dragging various sizes of oxygen containers. Then they become stronger and travel a short distance up Erwin Road to Duke Hospital for a lung transplant. A time of rejoicing at the Center is when these patients return without any supplemental oxygen and with a new look of hope in their eyes. After another 23 days, on an even happier occasion, many of these pulmonary rehab patients who have had lung transplants are able to return to their homes. Witnessing this life saving transformation has been a real blessing for me. And, and during this time I have been blessed to spend a good deal of time with my grandchildren, including trips with the older ones to Williamsburg and Jamestown. This opportunity, plus the many prayers that I know go up for me every day, gets me going each morning.

If I am fortunate enough to remain physically strong and active without a lung transplant for a while longer (only time will tell how long this may be since the prognosis for atypical IPF is unknown), my next goal is to do something to help publicize the little known IPF disease that kills as many people as breast cancer each year and has an overall survival rate of only one percent (those that receive a lung transplant). Motivated by Bob O'Rourke, a retired public relations person from Cal Tech and his recent program on NBC's Today Show, I would also like to become a spokesman for IPF and help raise research funds. Meanwhile, I am doing what I can to encourage my fellow patients at the Duke Pulmonary Rehab program.

Jim Clary can be contacted @: **jclary@mi-corporation.com**

*The Official Patient's Sourcebook on Idiopathic Pulmonary Fibrosis: A Revised and Updated Directory for the Internet Age by James N. Parker, M. D. and Philip M. Parker, PhD, Editors, published by ICON Health Publications, ICON Group International, Inc., San Diego, CA Copyright 2002*

"Idiopathic Pulmonary Fibrosis." It was published in *The Orphanet Journal of Rare Diseases* 2008, 3:8. The electronic version of this article can be found at www.ojrd.com/content/3/1/8

*American Journal of Respiratory Care Medicine,* Vol. 161, Number 2, February 2000, pp. 646-664 American Thoracic Society's publication, "Idiopathic Pulmonary Fibrosis: Diagnosis and Treatment: International Consensus Statement."

# From Collapse to Conquering

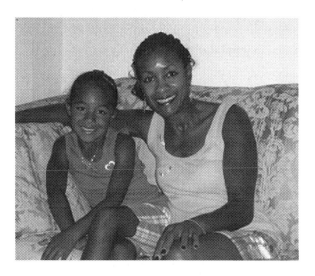

## *A Story of Brokenness and Bravery*

I have tried for 20 years to tell this story on paper. I hope that it will make a difference to someone. I have told it many times over the last 20 years yet I think it often carries no weight and the brush-off's are because each has his or her own life challenges and many are too busy to try to understand or too busy to care. My prayer is, if you are reading a book about pulmonary disease, that my story may be able to help you or someone you may know personally.

My story began in October of 1990. I was a young woman with a thriving life ahead of me, or so I thought. Around mid-October I began to not feel well. After a couple days of being ill, I decided to go to the emergency room to be checked out. There, I was given a prescription for antibiotics and released to go home. I believe the doctor just diagnosed my illness as a virus. I cannot be as definitive in my diagnosis and/or treatments as I would like to be without going through medical records. As I share more, you will understand why my doing that would be very challenging for me.

After my first emergency room visit, within the following two weeks there would be three more visits, each more severe than the prior, only because I was getting sicker and sicker. On Oct 24 or 25th of 1990, I made that fourth trip to the emergency room and barely made it out. I both entered and exited the emergency room visit in a wheelchair. Three or four days after that last emergency room trip also came what was almost the last day of my life. On Oct 29th, 1990, I had an appointment to see a physician at my local clinic. Before he ever examined me, he said two things to my family members that I recall, "First, she needs to be admitted to a hospital and secondly, she needs to be started on oxygen right away". My mother then drove me to the local hospital. I hardly remember getting admitted. I just remember struggling to get in and out of wheelchairs as I was transferred from clinics to cars to hospitals. I was admitted to the hospital. I recall the first time I had to use the bathroom I could not get out of the bed on my own. So I rang for a nurse to come to help me. The nurse stayed in the restroom with me and, as I was crying in pain, I recall her asking me, "What hurts?" or "Where was your pain?" I replied, "My back." She touched it or rubbed it to try relieving the pain. I remember screaming out loud, the last memory I have of that day but the beginning of many horrific memories ahead.

Writing such a long story in a limited amount of space is a challenge, and I cannot possibly go into detail about everything that happened. What I hope you'll gain from my story is the hope and inspiration that, no matter what you come up against in life, life is never over until it's over. God has the absolute final say in any situation. I know it was God who spared my life. The timing of being admitted to the hospital on the same day, and not only the same day, but hours before both of my lungs collapsed had to be God's grace.

Because both lungs collapsed, my heart also shifted. So, jokingly, I like to think that maybe it was not in the right place because my experience taught me how to live this life in a better way than I ever could have if this had not happened. From my understanding of what I have been told by others, a bleb burst inside of the lungs. When the air built up in the pleural space and was trapped in there (apparently my body was not absorbing the air), the pressure from the air that had built up in the pleural space caused the lungs to then collapse. This is called spontaneous pneumothorax. I don't recall all of the diagnoses that I've been given because they changed over the years, depending upon the problems I may have been experiencing at a specific time. I do recall some of my diagnoses, the first being A.R.D.S. Adult Respiratory Distress Syndrome. This was the first one that I can remember the physicians giving to my illness. I have also been given the diagnosis of Interstitial Lung Disease, and am currently carrying a diagnosis of bronchiectasis. Bronchiectasis is a condition in which damage to the airways causes them to widen and become flabby and scarred. The condition usually is the result of an infection or other occurrence that injures the walls of the airways, or, that prevents the airways from clearing mucus. I took this definition for Bronchiectasis from the internet to give it a proper definition. Now I would like to give it a personal definition by continuing to share my story and how it affects my life.

After my lungs collapsed, I can be nothing more than honest and say that I had a hell of a long road to travel ahead of me. I know that, in this world, we like to be positive and encouraging because there are so many negative factors that we have to face throughout each day. However, I will not and cannot share this story truthfully without sharing just how grim, dim, and bleak things looked many times throughout my ordeal. The positive and encouraging part to my story is that, 20 years later, I am still alive to share the same story. That should be enough to encourage anyone. If I don't tell how bad my nightmare was, then how can anyone enduring the same, or possibly worse, be encouraged?

I spent a lot of time in-patient, in many different hospital rooms from October, 1990, through December, 1991. I spent a total of nine and a half months of that time hospitalized. I did not have the "normal" hospital stay like most would think of a hospital stay. I was not able to get up and walk halls daily, use the bathrooms, eat or even have visitors, like most hospital patients. Because I was so sick, most of my stay was either in Intensive Care units or step down units which are operated by nurses that are specially trained to care for post-surgical patients. Actually, in a step down unit, the nurses' station is in the room with about 4 or 6 other patients. Because children tend to transmit germs often and more frequently than adults, I did not get to see my son on a regular basis. I was too critical most of the time. The doctors concerns were that I would become sicker if one of my visitors were ill.

After I was admitted to the hospital and my lungs collapsed, I found myself in intensive care for about 8 days, of which I don't have a lot of memory. I remember a few people hovering over my bed but not much else. I was probably too medicated or sedated to remember. I then was life-flighted to one of Pittsburgh's larger hospitals. There I would spend the rest of my residence hospital stays. I don't know how long a period of time passed before I woke after being air-lifted to Pittsburgh's Allegheny General Hospital, but, I recall awakening and realizing that the nightmare was not over yet. I was still sick and, at this point, in this very tiny room. Two nurses were in the room and one said to the other, "Everyone in this room dies". I came to grips with the reality that I could possibly and might very well be getting ready to leave this earth at the young age of 27. I was afraid of what was happening to me and what was going to be the outcome but I accepted the possibility of death.

I had a strong belief in God. Although I had not lived the godliest life, I believed in my faith enough to not fear an afterlife. I didn't want to die, though, because I felt that I had too much for which to live. I could not speak when I woke because I was intubated. I wondered if the nurses could sense my fears, my desperations, my neediness, and my unbreakable spirit that was soldiering for life. I can remember trying to show strength to everyone that I encountered. At the same time my show of strength was real, it also felt as though it was an act because, inside, I felt like breaking down some days, although never wanting to give up. I had days where I felt as though I could not take any more, even though I knew that I would fight to the end. I couldn't move, I was helpless, and totally dependent upon everyone else for my care, given my intubation, chest tubes, and IV's that connected me to all different types of machines, which made all sorts of noises around me day and night.

On December 8th, 1990, I had my first lung surgery. The doctors stated that I would come out of the surgery and have a couple of chest tubes, probably smaller than the ones that I had in and that I could be home by Christmas. They had to do the surgery because, in the six weeks that I had been hospitalized, chest tubes were not resolving the problem. Every time they pulled out one of the chest tubes, the lungs would collapse again. I came out of that surgery with 5 chest tubes, and I was released for the first time in February of 1991. I went home only to end up back in the hospital two weeks later, in March. I was in the hospital for about a month. I was released in April of 1991. I thought that I was taking it easy. I was even able to drive for a short while and resume a few light duties. All that came to an end around late June, 1991, when I began to feel fluid in my throat. I found myself coughing and spitting a lot. I noticed that the phlegm was mostly clear but I knew that something about it did not look right. There was white stuff in the middle of it and, at times, when I lay down, I had to quickly sit up because I felt as though I would choke on it.

In July, 1991, I was hospitalized again for a week. I was re-admitted because fluid had begun to build up in my chest, and the doctors did not know what the cause of it was. Different procedures were implemented and plenty of tests were run. But, when the team of physicians could not figure out what was the cause of it, I was informed that surgery was needed again to try and find a solution to the problem. One of the doctors told me that there was a good chance that I would not come through the surgery because I had just had the first surgery eight months prior. I was told by the doctor that I may want to say my good-byes. There was a part of me that knew the reality was that I could die, yet, in that reality I also knew that I was not going to go down without a fight.

I went in for that surgery and began another battle for my life. I ended up on the ventilator during most of this time and, after another long haul, I was released Christmas Eve, 1991. I then had to go through a year or so of recovery and, to this day, I still think of myself in a state of recovery. I will reiterate once again, the encouraging and inspirational part of my story is that, in 2011, I am still breathing and still functioning well enough to be able to continue to share my story with you, the reader.

I do plan on telling my story more detailed in full length, so please look for it sometime in the future or contact me to find out where I am at in the process: beecord@yahoo.com

# My Nightmare

Do you know what it's like not to be well
With parts of your body aching and swelled
Clumping and clotting all through your veins
Another shot of morphine to numb all your pain

Everyone tells you that you'll be ok
But you know your life could end this very day
Don't gag they say shoving tubes down your throat
No longer speaking communication by notes

Drawing blood in the morning taking pills in the night
Hallucination of witches and rituals of fright
You can't walk you can't stand you can't even sit up
And they're always asking you to urinate in a cup

Day in and day out you lie in a bed
Splints on your feet and you're almost dead
Depending on a machine no longer can you breathe
Your spirit is weary and ready to leave

Visions of people who you know are dead
Sneak in while you're sleeping and appear in your head
Please someone help me this must be a dream
Take this tube out of my throat so that I can please scream

Prepped for surgery to go under the knife
Being told possibly that you'll lose your life
Fevers a burning temperatures high
Seeing the troubles look in your loved ones eyes

A tear rolls down from the corner of your eye
It's time to go in now please say good bye
Bright shining lights are glowing in your face
It's time to go to sleep now your heart starts to race

Awakening to darkness adjusting to light
Machine still breathing for me my lungs are too tight
Tubes in my sides and each of my ends
Wanting and needing the hand of a friend

Not wanting to live and not wanting to die
Questioning and praying and always asking why
Month after month and room after room
I need to get out of here to go home real soon

The old year has gone the new one has come
I'm still in this hospital away from my son

*Beverly Cordes*

# Surviving Lung Cancer

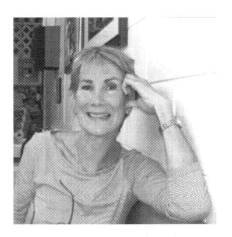

## *A Story of a Journey Within*

*"Go home tonight and write a theme and let that theme come out of you and then it will be true . . . ."*

The coincidence of seeing Langston Hughes' poem "Theme for English B" framed on the wall of Duke's Morris Cancer Clinic stopped me in my tracks. It's a poem about a teacher assigning her students to write down their stories. I was there on my way to an initial meeting with the Chief of Thoracic Surgery. Over the years I had assigned this very poem as an effective writing ice-breaker, a tool to draw out the personal stories in the Developmental English class I taught at Butner Federal Prison. As I made my way to my appointment, I reflected that I was the one doing time now waiting for a verdict on my health. This time the poem seemed to be asking the teacher what story would come out of her tonight!

Despite the snow storm that had delivered a one-two punch to my southern city that winter, I managed to secure the CD composite of follow-up scans from Durham Radiology. These scans were something that my doctor agreed hadn't changed perceptibly in four years. That disc was my evidence for this meeting with the new big deal doctor that lung surgery was not warranted and I clutched it tightly. But I was worried. I had dodged the bullet so far and, after my terror facing the dragon of my mortality after the first scan, I had convinced myself that the "small nodule" in my right lung was scar tissue from a bout with pneumonia in my twenties some forty years ago. The many follow-up CT and PET scans didn't disavow me of this notion and over the years, I came to take the scans in stride. I just needed the new doctor to see things my way. "This doctor has skills I don't have", my near—retirement doctor told me in a hand-off meeting in January following a PET scan. "I think he's going to want to do surgery", he added quietly, as I was leaving the office.

My story actually began four years earlier, in 2006. It had a benign enough a beginning—routine annual physical with my Internist of 10 years. I typically had nothing to report at this meeting. I was born a few months short of being classified a baby boomer. Like many in that generation, I played hard, worked hard, and I ate mindfully. I also took no medications and hadn't smoked for 30 years. But this time, I casually mentioned having a dry cough for a couple weeks. The month was October, and the pollen and the leaf spores were part and parcel of doing my own yard work, I offered helpfully to the doctor, hoping this was the real issue, allergies. My father's death from lung cancer in his 60's was part of my medical record, however, and this fact was not lost in my long relationship with this doctor. "But he was a fireman," I added, "occupational hazard!". "A fireman who smoked, as you did, for 15 years", she countered. "Let's get a chest scan."

The book, *The Warmth of Other Suns,* was on the best seller list the year I found out I had lung cancer. The title was a line from a Richard Wright poem telling of his long ago escape from the oppression of the South. I thought about the irony of my escape *to* the South 13 years before! My retired husband, Pat, and I, too were seeking the 'warmth of other suns' after 16 snowfalls fell on our Chatham, N.J. home that winter. We put our house on the market and began exploring some southern cities. The South was unknown territory to us. So, with the help of Money Magazine's endorsement of the Triangle as one of the "Best Places to Live" that year, we began our search and ultimately chose Durham, N.C. Years would pass before either Durham's reputation as the 'City of Medicine', or the irony of Durham's and my tobacco heritage would come into play in my life. Back then, Joe Camel billboards still dotted Highway 501, the route our moving truck took to our new sunny location.

So what's with all this snow this year, I wondered as I made my way through the corridors of the Morris Clinic. As I waited with fragile confidence that day, an upbeat PA prepared me for the meeting with the doctor. She had seen my records and heard my defense, and volunteered that she agreed I was probably not a candidate for surgery at that time. But the doctor tricked us that day. He listened so intently to my defense that I thought I had won him over. But then, as if he hadn't heard me at all, he said calmly, "You have a 60-40 chance of cancer." Or did he say 40-60? Whatever the order of his words, they had the force of a stun gun. I didn't like these numbers. They weren't low enough or high enough to help me out of the deep freeze I suddenly entered. There wasn't enough wiggle room in those odds, or air in the room. When I next heard him say "If you were my wife . . .", my defenses melted and a tear fell down my face. The scenario was like an episode from a Groucho Marks' show where the contestant said the magic word. The night before I had this goofy thought that if the doctor offered, "If you were my wife", I'd know what I had to do. I never figured him to say so personal a statement because I had Googled him and he was much younger than I and a chief surgeon! My husband suggested that I sleep on it, but I declined. The day of reckoning had come.

The operation was scheduled for three weeks hence, February 26, 2010. I experienced a state of grace that first week which, in hindsight, could have been a state of shock. I told the people I wanted to know. I cried a little. I researched lung studies a little. This organ that I had taken for granted, to my surprise, had five lobes. (I had thought four). The right lung had three lobes and my problem node was in the upper right. I didn't know what to make of two different X-ray technicians who commented during pre-op that I had long lungs but their statement made me hopeful that the length could somehow make up for the missing volume. Week two before surgery, I met the devil. The fear that crept into my bedroom in the night was oppressive. It took over my whole being and robbed me of my peace, my sleep, and my appetite. I wrestled it for several days and wondered how I would survive until the operation. My husband worried for me and cared for me but could bring little relief from my suffering. I was back in the dilemma of the numerical probability of having cancer. I wanted to cancel the operation or have it immediately.

The doctor's office had no cancellations and his PA had little patience for my terror. I resorted to begging a sleeping potion from a neighbor for a night's sleep but the sorry-state Joan who went to sleep that night was still waiting for me in the morning. In this lost state, a paper titled "A Cup of Trembling" came to mind. The title seemed to describe my physical condition. A new friend had presciently urged me to read this paper the previous summer. It was a treatise on suffering, and I now wondered if I could put my hands on it. I located it easily, to my surprise, in a reading stack in my bedroom and placed it, unread, on the bed. My immediate concern was a birthday dinner scheduled for my husband at our club that night. I knew I couldn't fake celebration. The thought of food and forced conversation nauseated me. I presented my sorry self to my husband that morning and devised a plan. I would excuse myself early in the dinner, before the food came, and I would go home, offering some excuse by cell for my absence. But, a couple hours before the party, still miserable, I sadly realized how far off track I had gotten.

Like Christian in the *Pilgrims Progress,* my favorite allegory, who had wandered off the Path and was captured by the Giant

Despair, I too, found myself in a dark dungeon in Doubting Castle. In the book, Christian, realizing his mistake, begins to pray. He remembers the key in his bosom called Promise that can open any door in Doubting Castle. That afternoon, reading "The Cup of Trembling" was the little key that set me free. I prayed and read the paper. I then contemplated, first Job's suffering, and next Christ's suffering in Gethsemane, an event so mesmerizing I read as if for the first time and surrendered myself again to the One who first called me his own. When I finished my meditation, I realized that I was transformed. My fear was gone completely! I tested it with all manner of imaginings. My appetite returned and I had great enthusiasm for the celebration ahead. I had experienced a miracle. And I celebrated with abandon that night. This touch from God would carry me to and through the dark days of surgery and recovery.

I recall my hospital experience as three days in the belly of the whale! The surgeon had prepared me that a biopsy during surgery would dictate whether I would need to have a lobectomy. Ever hopeful, I was surprised to wake up hours later minus a lobe. Sleep would be elusive. In my little corner room, I stared at the clock through all the watches of the night. I begged for one hour of sleep. The continuous noise and pressure of the air filled equipment on my legs tortured me and I finally prevailed on a nurse to remove them. I pressed the pain button reluctantly during the nights not knowing I couldn't overdose with it. But sleep wouldn't come until six a.m., just as the chirpy interns made their rounds. The food trays came and went untouched. Nausea ruled. Absent food, I vomited bile. Weak, yet determined to get out in three days, I obediently walked the floor around and around, my head spinning from the drugs. Three pounds lighter the eve of day two, blessed relief came when a new nurse placed a little round patch behind my right ear. In two hours, my nausea was gone. I had never been on a cruise or in the belly of a whale, and didn't know to ask for nausea relief. That night the little room closed in on me, and I had a panic attack. Visiting hours were over so I called my praying friend who talked me down. I had a scare day three when I was told the terms of leaving the hospital that day. I had to have a bowel movement. That was ludicrous! There had not been any garbage in to get the garbage out! In three days, I had consumed only one bowl of my husband's homemade chicken broth with noodles. I wondered what the chances were of those scant noodles finding their way out by three o'clock. But, the compassionate nurse had some medical tricks up her sleeve and I was able to leave the hospital that day.

This month is a year since my surgery. I will have an important scan soon. I've learned that cancer, even if 'they get it all", still has some power to haunt me, like something that goes bump in the night. I've also learned that healing is relative. My healing is taking much longer than my optimistic, impatient self thought. I gave myself two months to be back on my feet. After all, the green book on preparing for lung surgery said I could be driving in two months. I adjusted my thinking monthly after that goal was missed. At four months, I asked to see my surgeon about a persistent, debilitating cough that made my friends ask, "What's with that?" I coughed whenever I spoke and soon stopped talking. Five more pounds had slipped off my bony frame from lack of sleep and appetite. The doctor agreed to schedule me for a 24 day course of pulmonary rehab at Duke's Center for Living that I had heard about from a neighbor. I apparently fell into some sorry statistic of six percent who present such coughing symptoms after surgery.

The Center for Living provided many things besides a destination three days a week to build back up. I was not alone there. I was assigned to the pulmonary group and, in time, decrypted the color charts we each were assigned. Yellow meant waiting for transplant; blue, post-transplant. I was green—other. There was no room on the exercise floor for self-pity. Unlike me, most of the participants were carting oxygen. I exercised alongside hopeful veterans of pain and suffering, many a long way from the comforts of home. There I learned the anatomy of the lung and how and why to breath properly using my diaphragm. Over time, during the monotonous rhythms of the floor exercises, I reflected on the gratitude I felt for my life, and gratitude for my doctors: the referring ones and the surgeon bold enough to suggest surgery. I was grateful to this doctor who was skilled enough to remove the cancer, leaving only two barely perceptible scars. I gave thanks too for the caring Physical Therapy staff. On the gym floor, I let the faces of those who visited me, vacuumed, brought food, flowers, birdseed, healing books, tapes and cards come before me. One even mowed my grass, a job to which I longed to get back. My sister sent a lemon tree from California with a note, "When life gives you lemons! . . ." I especially treasured the prayer quilt the ladies at Duke Chapel made for me, each hand tied knot representing a prayer.

"There is no agony like bearing an untold story inside you", the main character in Zora Hurston's book, *Their Eyes Were Watching God,* remarks. So I am grateful to get my story out for this writing project. The seed was planted a year ago in the Morris Clinic with the poem's line, "Go home tonight and write a theme and let that theme come out of you . . ." It germinated at the Center for Living. Difficult as it has been to revisit some of these places, the writing has been a healing exercise and a blessing. My progress is apparent. The first thing most people notice is that my cough is practically gone. Then they'll comment that I'm looking well, which translates that I've finally put on some weight. I walk two to three miles a day now, summer and winter, without a mask. With each day, and as the time of my scan approaches, I draw comfort in the words of the mystic, Julian of Norwich, *"All shall be well and all shall be well and all manner of things shall be well."*

Joan K. Zax

# Being Diagnosed With COPD Saved My Life

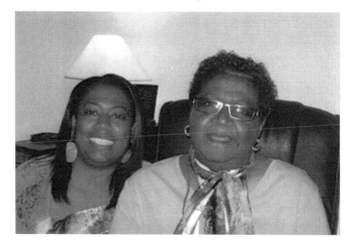

## *A Story about Moving Forward with the Challenges of Life*

My name is Shirley White and I currently live with a disease called COPD, (Chronic Obstructive Pulmonary Disease). I purposely said "live with" because I am a testimony of what to do and what not to do concerning lung disease. Prior to moving to Durham, North Carolina, in 2002, I had lived in Atlantic City, New Jersey, all of my life. As a former smoker, I never imagined my life would turn out the way it did. I was never a heavy smoker, and, I hardly drank alcohol, so I thought I was living a somewhat healthy life. Right around the time the government started really cracking down on tobacco companies and forcing them to share the dangers associated with smoking, I was diagnosed with asthma. I immediately quit that terrible habit but more health issues came along years down the road. Shortly after retiring from the Atlantic City Medical Center in the mid 1990s where I worked as a Dietary Technician, my asthma condition worsened. I'd like to think my condition got worse because I was no longer being active but the reasons are not clear.

As my condition worsened, using oxygen was suggested when I felt short of breath, and, I was placed on a Bi-Pap machine after failing a sleep study test. I was diagnosed with Sleep Apnea, which was somewhat scary to me. I lived at home with my youngest child, an active one who stayed on the go, so, for the most part, I was home alone. I knew I felt tired a lot of the time and my son would find me sleeping at the kitchen table, but I never thought it was due to sleep apnea. What a scary disease.

I'm scared to think that, while I was sleeping, I actually stopped breathing for periods of time. In the beginning, I did my best to wear the head gear that comes with the Bi-Pap machine. It truly takes some getting used to. Sometimes I would take a break from it when I felt my lungs were strong enough. I tried to manage my disease, which I later realized wasn't such a good idea. After going so many nights without using the Bi-Pap machine, weeks or even sometimes months down the line, I would end up in the hospital due to breathing complications. This would happen once or twice a year. I realized that my illness was something I would have to live with for the rest of my life. This realization still didn't make the mask any more comfortable and I would still cheat even though I knew deep down inside that I was hurting myself. With all that was going on in my life, I still tried to live a fulfilled life after retirement. Several times a year I would visit my daughters who lived in Durham and I would vacation with my youngest once a year. During one of my visits, I had one of my episodes where I had difficulty breathing. I knew I wasn't feeling myself but I didn't want to bother anyone. I was 500 miles away from my doctor. I felt that, if I could only hold out until I get back home, I should be okay. My daughter came home from work, only to find me in the same place she left me that morning.

She told me that I was shaking and that I was going in and out of consciousness. She called the ambulance that took me to Duke Hospital. I was extremely anxious, because I didn't know what to expect from these strangers. The doctors were not familiar with me nor my health issues, so I was concerned about how they were to treat me effectively. Once they got my breathing under control, they told me that my calcium was low, and that I was suffering from anxiety. I had never been diagnosed with either of these conditions. I was given something to increase my calcium level while in the hospital emergency room, and I was prescribed a muscle relaxer for the anxiety. I was released from the emergency room and I went back home with my daughter. I was a little disoriented still from the muscle relaxers. I had never taken them before, so I wasn't sure how they were going to make me feel. The next thing I remember I was back at the hospital. My daughter told me that I appeared to have gone into a very deep sleep because of the muscle relaxers and, at some point, had stopped breathing. This trip to the emergency room was very different from the day before. As I went in and out of consciousness, I remember being scared because I knew this time it was something very serious. I guess a couple days had gone by before I woke up to see that I was on a ventilator.

I had been on a ventilator once before while in the hospital up in New Jersey, but there was something different this time. I was told that my carbon dioxide level was dangerously high and they were having trouble trying to control it. After 3 or 4 days, they took me off of the ventilator, and my carbon dioxide level shot back up through the roof. The doctors came into my room and told me that I was very ill. My daughters were all at work, so I had to receive this information alone. I was told that I had a chronic case of COPD and that I needed surgery ASAP. They called my youngest daughter with whom I had been staying, Cassandra (Sam) Adkins, and gave her the news. Here I was, miles away from home and about to undergo a very serious surgery. The surgery they recommended was called a Tracheotomy. I was scared before, but I was beyond scared this time. My world as I knew it was about to change forever. Other than giving birth, I had never had any other major procedure done. For the first time in my life I felt alone and terrified. What was going to become of my life? How could I face the world or my family with a hole in my neck? The way I talk was going to change. People will begin to look at me strangely and talk behind my back.

Before I was released from the hospital, my three sons and the grand-daughter I raised now with a newborn all came to Durham to see the new me. The procedure was a success, and all those fears I had weren't as bad as I thought. My life changed, but at least I still had life. Without the love and support of my children, I don't know how I could have gone through this. They would show me time and time again, that I had so much to live for and that I should fight. So that is what I did. We decided that I should stay with my daughter, Sam, in Durham and not go back to New Jersey. My daughter and I often talked about my moving in with her since she was a little girl.

A mother always wants to see her children grow up and move on with their own lives, have children, and become productive citizens. But here I was at the young age of 67 and my independence was about to take a drastic turn. Even though we always talked about it, I wasn't quite ready to be taken care of and I'm not so sure that my daughter was ready. As a mother, one never wants to become a burden on one's children. In order for this to work, I knew I would have to stay strong and try to maintain the lifestyle that I was used to living. I've always done my own cooking, cleaning, shopping, bathing, and paying of bills. I hoped to keep on doing these things, maybe with a little help only when needed.

A month had passed since I got my trach and I was going to the clinic at Duke to have it changed. Before leaving the hospital, the doctors went back and forth on what kind of trach I needed. They tried the metal trach. Later I had complications with it so I ended up being released with a cuffed trach. My daughters have all been trained on how to care for my trach but, Sam, my primary caregiver, has become quite the pro on trach care. She has taken up shop right next to the hospital bed in which I now sleep. She does all the suctioning and does a great job at keeping the trach clean. Being that this is still fairly new to both of us, the doctors and therapist thought it would be best that I go to the clinic to have the trach changed versus having someone come out to do it at my home. My first visit didn't go as well as I had hoped. While in the hospital, the therapist did had some trouble getting the cuffed trach in, though nothing like I experienced at the clinic. Nothing could have prepared me for what I was about to go through. The doctors weren't even prepared for what happened. Everything was going fine until the nurse tried to pull out the trach and couldn't. Soon they had to call for backup because the nurse wasn't able to do it by herself. The sight of all those white coats ran my pressure through the roof. Within minutes I was being whisked off to the hospital. I don't remember much but what I do remember wasn't pleasant. When they attempted to pull the trach out, the skin at the opening of the trach was torn. Fearing the blood would get into my lungs, they sent me over to the hospital to complete the procedure. My blood pressure went up along with my carbon dioxide. I ended up having to stay in the hospital for a couple days. The same thing happened the following month when I went in to have my trach changed. Out of the six or so times I went to the clinic, four of those times I ended up at the hospital. The doctors soon realized that they had to come up with another method for switching out the trach each month. I've been maintaining good care throughout the month as, again, my daughter has been doing a great job keeping the area clean and free from infection. They decided to switch me over to a cuffed-less trach and that seemed to be the answer to all of our prayers. Going through the procedure each month was hard for me but just as hard for the doctors and nurses. To sum it up, we weren't able to find a good rhythm in changing the trach each month. We just didn't know what to expect. Life with the cuffed-less trach was improved. We have finally found our stride. My daughter (the pro) was trained on how to change the trach and she has been able to do it at home once a month without any problems. My pressure stays at a reasonable level and I'm in the comfort of my own home. All of these factors have really made a big difference in my confidence and willingness to go on. I don't know how much more I could have taken going to the clinic each month, only to be admitted into the hospital. Coming off the cuffed trach also meant I no longer needed to sleep with a ventilator. Hallelujah!!!!

Life has truly been great over the last several years. While I was going through all the ups and downs with my trach, I also started a class at the Duke Center for Living. Going there also helped build my confidence and strengthened my willingness to live. Never in my life had I done exercise. Here I am in my late 60s going to a class 3 days a week. For the first time ever, I have developed muscles in places I couldn't have imagined. I look forward to going to the Center every week. The therapist and staff are all so nice and helpful. What has surprised me the most are the friendships I have developed. A good relationship is the one with someone that's going through similar health issues. We check up on each other and we look out for each other. This is something I'm not used to but I welcomed it with open arms. Everyone genuinely cares about the next person and we all want the best for each other. To see a fellow patient fight through his or her illness encourages me to do the same. In the end, we all get better and we are all grateful for the love and support that is expressed throughout the Duke Center for Living. The center has truly made a difference in my life because, each time I have a setback, I'm able to go back to the Center and rebuild my strength and will to live. I think that's why they named it "The Center for Living"

Living with COPD, I have good days and bad days. Thank God, most of my days have been good days. I sometimes get a little down when I think about how my life used to be. I miss the condo I had while living in New Jersey. I miss the freedom I felt and, deep down inside, I miss being a mother. Now my children are caring for me instead of my caring for them. I sometimes get angry when I feel I have no control over my life and I'm expected to do what they think is best for me. Sometimes I want to boycott. Sometimes I want to yell and scream, "You are not my mother!!". I know my daughters mean well and they have my best interest at heart but giving up everything is hard when I'm so used to being the one in control. I believe what I feel at times is depression, something one doesn't want to think or even admit one might be suffering. So I push my way through it until I feel good about myself and my situation. Dealing with the feelings can be very draining because one keeps what he or she truly is feeling to one's self. What have I done in my lifetime to deserve this outcome? What could I have done different to change my situation? I don't know if I'll ever be 100% okay with how things turned out but I have learned to make the very best of my situation. Again, my good days outweigh the bad, and I'm thankful for my family and the love and support of friends. I couldn't imagine going through all I've gone through alone. My situation has even drawn me closer to God, never a bad thing. I go to church with my daughters now, something of which I never dreamed. I'm so thankful now to have such memories. When I think about the experience, my quality of life is better than I could have imagined. I've been able to travel out of the country, another something of which I never even dreamed. My whole life was contained in New Jersey with an occasional bus trip to a different state to shop. Then I ended up in North Carolina. Now my life has taken a turn such as this. I now want to live and experience all that life has to offer. I will admit that life gets scary sometimes but one has to learn to make lemonade with lemons. With this type of illness, one is susceptible to other diseases, and I have had my fair share of them. My stays at Duke Hospital are never pleasant but at least I've been able to leave under my own will. At one time, there was a push for me to lose between 120-150 lbs, because they wanted to reverse the tracheotomy procedure. People don't normally live with a trach. They are intended to be a temporary solution. I've been living with my trach for almost nine years now. They no longer talk to me about reversing the procedure because this is what has been working for me. As long as I do my part by trying to eat right, exercise, and follow the instructions from my doctors, I believe God will add many more years to my life. I live a very abundant life at 75 years young, as I just had another grandchild born a year ago. The list of great-grands continues to grow as well, and I love them all. Family is what keeps me going. During my darkest times, it was my family that pulled me through, spiritually and sometimes even physically. One can live with a lung disease and one can live a very fulfilled life. I am a living testimony.

*Shirley White*

# *But you don't look sick . . . .*

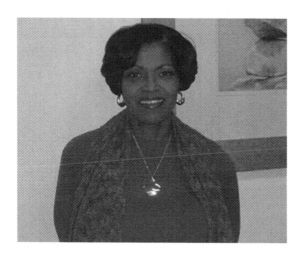

## *A Story of a Unique Disease*

In 1983, while finishing my senior year of nursing at UNC-Chapel Hill, I began to have difficulty breathing through my nose and I was experiencing episodes of shortness of breath. I was on top of the world. I had attended the college of my dreams, the University of North Carolina at Chapel Hill, made good grades, and fulfilled a dream that I had since childhood to work in the medical field helping others. I finished my course work in four years and had excelled at UNC as a single parent and adult student.

After graduation, I was hired as a registered nurse in the surgical intensive care unit. I was so excited about this job and was ready to make my mark in critical care nursing. The job was very stressful because I cared for patients with life-threatening illnesses. Little did I know that this stress would intensify the symptoms I was having and lead to a diagnosis of Sarcoidosis. The following information was taken from (http://www. stopsarcoidosis.org/sarcoidosis/diseasefacts.htm )

Sarcoidosis (pronounced SAR-COY-DOE-SIS) is an inflammatory disease that can affect almost any organ in the body. It causes heightened immunity, which means that a person's immune system, which normally protects the body from infection and disease, overreacts, resulting in damage to the body's own tissues. The disease can go into remission without medical intervention. It can also flare up during periods of stress.

Sarcoidosis most commonly affects the lungs and lymph nodes, but the disease can and usually does affect others organs, too, including (but not limited to) the skin, eyes, liver, salivary glands, sinuses, kidneys, heart, the muscles and bones, and the brain and nervous system. It can also cause "cognitive fog", where you just can't seem to think clearly. Sarcoidosis is now known to be common and affects people worldwide. The disease can affect people of any age, race and gender. However, it is most common among adults between the ages of 20 and 40 and in certain ethnic groups. In the United States, it is most common in African-Americans and people of European descent, particularly those from Scandinavia. African Americans are the most affected U.S. group. Their estimated lifetime risk of developing Sarcoidosis might be as high as two percent. Most studies suggest an even higher disease rate for women.

I didn't see a doctor until September, 1984. I was 33 years old, and I thought I was a healthy, energetic, athletic, mature woman who was on top of the world. I just had difficulty breathing. My sinuses and head ached all the time and I had periodic episodes of shortness of breath. The doctor I initially saw misdiagnosed me as having allergies. Another told me I was stressed and needed to calm down. So I made an appointment with an allergist and was tested and learned that grasses and trees were the culprits. I began immunotherapy for the allergies. But, my sinus problems continued to worsen and the shortness of breath intensified. I went to an ENT surgeon, and he found that I had a deviated septum, which he said could be corrected by surgery. It was after this surgery that my surgeon said, "Miss Barnette, your pathology report says you have Sarcoidosis", I'm sorry". I was puzzled as to why he said he was sorry. Many years later I understood why he said he was sorry—my life would never be the same once I was diagnosed with Sarcoidosis. When the surgeon removed the sarcoid growth/granulomas, the operation created an open wound that would never heal and one that would always be susceptible to infection.

At the time, I had no other symptoms of Sarcoidosis, so I was given steroid nasal spray and told to rinse my nose three times a day with salt water. This ritual controlled the drainage for a while, but in 1988, my nose became very inflamed with infection. I sought the help of an Infectious Disease doctor who specialized in treating patients with Sarcoidosis. Cultures were obtained, and they found that I had staphylococcus growing in my nose. Antibiotics were ordered and My health improved.

A pulmonary function test began a 12 year journey of increased symptoms of Sarcoidosis in my lungs, and I was prescribed many medications. I experienced episodes of wheezing and shortness of breath. So my doctor put me on prednisone, a drug that is commonly prescribed as a treatment for a flare-up of Sarcoidosis. It decreased the inflammation in my lungs, but the side effects were dreadful. I couldn't sleep, I gained weight and my face changed to a moon face. No one recognized me! The mood swings and personality changes were the worst. My bones began to break and I ended up with fractures in both feet and a stress fracture in my left leg. These fractures took a very long time to heal since prednisone slows down the healing process.

In addition to the weight gain, I began to get more infections in my nose. One culture result was particularly worrisome. I had contracted MRSA (methicillin resistant staphylococcus). This infection was serious! Only one antibiotic existed, Vancomycin®, that would kill this bacteria and it would not treat the infection if I took it by mouth. I had to have a Hickman catheter inserted into one of the main vessels that led to my heart. This was necessary since Vancomycin® is a very strong antibiotic and giving it in any other vein would damage my veins permanently. I took this drug for approximately six weeks. After 3 months the catheter was removed and I improved. But, because I was still on steroids the MRSA returned, another Hickman was inserted about a year later. It was a revolving door of infections and antibiotics.

In July of 1997, I began having severe, stabbing unilateral facial pain that was triggered by touching or pressing on areas on my face or back of my neck. It started with a sensation of electric shocks to my right temple and then built up to an excruciating pain felt deep in my head. The pain would fade away in an hour to be replaced by a burning ache that lasted hours. Many diagnoses and medications were given but nothing eliminated the headache. My ENT doctor ordered a MRI and found that I had significant Sarcoidosis granulomas in my middle ear. We thought we had identified the culprit that was causing the pain. I was scheduled for a mastoidectomy of my right ear in November of 1997 that surgically removed the growths in the bone behind the ear (mastoid bone), including removal of the anvil, hammer and stapes of the middle ear. Its purpose is to create a "safe" ear and prevent further damage to the hearing apparatus. I prayed that this surgery would stop those awful headaches and, for a time, I did not have any really bad headaches. But they came back in 2002 and I was devastated because no one could tell me why I was having these excruciating headaches. The neurologist I saw was extremely rude and would doubt my description of the pain. I finally found an anesthesiologist who diagnosed me with trigeminal neuralgia. He felt that I may have sarcoid granulomas on my trigeminal nerve and they were causing irritation which was leading to these awful headaches.

During this time I learned how society treats people who are obese. I didn't look sick; I looked like I had no discipline about eating. I was ridiculed on airplanes about the amount of space I was taking in the seat. People looked at me and shook their heads. Friends and family did not recognize me. I began to isolate myself and only go to work, church and home.

It is difficult to face a chronic illness every day that affects your ability to breath. You wake up, it's there. You go to bed at night, it's there. But sometimes you just have to play the hand you're dealt!

God reminded me that everyone can't suffer. I read scriptures on healing; I prayed; I had others pray for me. Every day I thanked God for healing me. I prayed for others to be healed. I taught others about God's healing power, even though I had not recovered or seen the evidence of healing in my own life. I just had faith, the Bible states in Hebrews 11:1 "Now faith is the substance of things hoped for, the evidence of things not seen" (King James Version, Cambridge Edition). I knew that God's word was true and that I would be healed. I just didn't know when. I had to exercise that faith muscle daily until I became stronger and stronger and my belief put joy in my heart. Contentment replaced the anxiety I always felt. A joy came to me about the simple things of life and just admiring His creation put me at peace even though everything around me was falling apart.

In January 2004 I tried once again to get off the prednisone without having a "flare up" which would require an increase of the steroids rather than a decrease. I decided to pray and ask God to show me how to taper the drug so as not to cause a flare up. I found that I could trick my body by very slowly taking the dosage down a milligram every week. If I had symptoms, I would stay on that dosage another week. It took me until September, 2004, to completely take myself off Prednisone. I continued to take Methotrexate which is a prednisone sparing drug.

My lungs stayed clear as long as I didn't get sick. I steer clear of people who are sick or who are coughing. I don't play with young children without washing my hands. I use precautions when around people who are smoking, (cigarette smoke triggers a flare up). Also, I've noticed that when I am extremely stressed,

I have more symptoms with my skin. I have since retired from my job in 2006 and that seemed to really help my stress level.

The journey continues but not as intense. My lung function has improved and my doctors say my lung function is normal.

I've lost 200lbs; I can exercise with minimal pain, I eat right and read my Bible to stay spiritually strong. I feel that I have been restored and that God " . . . *has renewed my youth like the eagles".* Psalms 103:5 (King James Version, Cambridge Edition).

*Virginia M. Barnette*

References

"FSR—Sarcoidosis Disease Facts & Statistics." *Foundation for Sarcoidosis Research.* Web. 24 Feb. 2011. <http://www.stopsarcoidosis.org/sarcoidosis/diseasefacts.htm

"Kevin Ho Ear Nose and Throat—San Francisco." *San Francisco Ear Nose & Throat Specialist—Dr. Kevin Ho.* Web. 24 Feb. 2011. <http://www.kevinhomd.com/Mastoid.html>.

The Holy Bible

# THE COMMAND TO
# BECOME A CAREGIVER

# How I Loved My Mother to Life

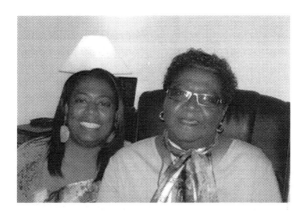

*A Story of a Daughter along with her Siblings and the Love They Share for Their Mother*

My mother, Shirley White, came from Atlantic City, N.J., to visit me here in Durham, N.C., during the summer of 2002. Since her retirement in the mid-1990's, her sleep apnea seemed to worsen, but not to the point where it prevented her from traveling and doing the things that she loved. I also have two sisters that live here in Durham, and we all love getting together to go out to the movies and going to Walmart. As far as I knew, she was using her bi-pap as recommended and things were under control. While visiting with me, we enjoyed each other's company and nothing appeared to be out of the ordinary.

I came home from work one day for lunch to find my mother shaking. I called the ambulance and she was rushed her to the hospital. At that time, I was told her calcium was low and that she suffered from anxiety. They gave her something for the calcium and some muscle relaxers for the anxiety and sent her home. When we got home, my mother seemed to go into a deep sleep. I thought it was the medicine she had just received while at the hospital so I wasn't too concerned. But as I kept watch, I noticed a change in her breathing. I dialed 911 again and she was rushed back to the hospital. This time she was barely conscious. Her carbon dioxide (blood gas) level was 106, which is extremely high. This time I wasn't able to take her back home with me because she was admitted into Duke's ICU. She was placed on a breathing machine to assist with getting her gas level back to normal.

After three or four days, her blood gas level dropped down to 75, and she was taken off of the ventilator. The doctor said she must use her bi-pap machine every night, and also recommended that she lose weight. The next day her blood gas began going up and down so they recommended that she use the bi-pap 24 hours a day. She didn't like that news but agreed that it was the best option at the time. She was willing to do anything so she could go home. While at work the following week, I got a phone call from a Dr. Clay at Duke stating that he wanted to proceed with a tracheotomy. Her blood gas level continued to fluctuate from day to day, hour to hour, and her doctors felt the time had come to consider other options concerning her survival. The doctors said that if they didn't move forward with the procedure soon, my mother would die. Her gas level had jumped up to 115, which is higher than the initial reading when first admitted into ICU.

I'll never forget that day. It was on Wednesday, September 4, 2002. After I got myself together, I called my brothers and sisters and gave them the grave news. We all realized that this was a life or death decision, and without hesitation, we chose life for our mother. They put her back on the ventilator and scheduled the surgery for Friday. This is when our new journey began.

As a little girl, I always knew that, one day, my mother would come to live with me. Recently divorced, I had just purchased a new home the previous year. During my search I made sure that

I had room for my mother. I had no idea that her coming to stay with me would happen so soon after getting my home, but I was okay with it. While living in New Jersey, my mother lived alone. After getting the news about my mother's need for a trach, as a family we decided that her staying with me was best, I became her primary care provider. My mother was finally diagnosed as having COPD, Chronic Obstructive Pulmonary Disease. Given all the physical therapy, speech therapy, trying to figure out what kind of trash to use, what size trach to use, and what would be the best aftercare, she must have stayed in the hospital three or four weeks. My sisters and I met with the Apria Aftercare team. We were trained on how to operate the ventilator machine, how to suction her, how to give her breathing treatments, and how to clean around the trach.

At the end of her stay at Duke, God gave us a brand new mother. She was 30 pounds lighter and she looked great! I went out and purchased a twin air mattress and a baby monitor. We moved the bed that was in the downstairs bedroom upstairs and replaced it with a hospital bed. For months, I slept beside my mother's bed on the air mattress. As soon as the alarm went off on the ventilator, I was right there, ready to execute all of my training. For the most part, my mother is very easy going so it didn't take much for her to adapt to her new home and lifestyle. She was still around family with all three of her daughters living here in Durham, N.C., and my three brothers would come down to visit at least three or four times a year from N.J. I very quickly became a pro at suctioning her and cleaning around her trach.

Also, as part of her discharge, she was to begin attending an exercise class at the Duke Center for Living. Mom isn't an outgoing person, so, to get her involved in an exercise class was difficult. But, she knew doing so is what would keep her alive. She was willing to do it. Back in N.J., my mother had just two or three former co-workers with whom she stayed in touch and she hardly went out of the house. She was always quiet and kept to herself. So, for her to be involved with something where she would be surrounded by strangers was a very big deal. Though she had a slow start because everything was so new to her, she did not take too long to get into the swing of things.

After a few weeks, she started looking forward to going to the Duke Center for Living, where they specialize in the rehabilitation of patients with respiratory conditions of all kinds. After a few more weeks, she would come home and tell me stories about the friends that she had made. For the first time in my life, I saw a different side to my mother. I saw a more outgoing person, a more compassionate person, and a person with a new found desire to live. After she completed the initial four to five week class, she began going three days a week. She would get herself together each of those mornings like she was getting prepared to go to a job, so, I began calling this routine her job. Instead of getting a paycheck, she is getting added years to her life. Things have been going well for the both of us. I was able to get back to a normal work schedule, and my mother had her weekly schedule at the Center for Living. I was working for IBM at the time. My superiors were very understanding when I had to take time off to care for my mother. I was allowed to work a flex schedule so that I could take her to each of her doctor appointments. Things were going quite well at home. Each month, we had to go into the Duke Clinic to have her cuffed trach tube changed. Every time her trach tube had to be changed there would be complications because the balloon on the tube would rip at the opening. It would tear the skin when they pulled the trach tube out, which made her very anxious and caused her blood pressure to go up. On at least three occasions we went from the clinic to the hospital. Her vitals would get so out of control that she would get admitted directly into the ICU unit where she would be safe and they had all the necessary equipment available to treat her. Her doctors realized that changing this particular kind of trach tube was putting too much stress on her body and decided to switch her over to a cuff-less trach tube. Things changed from that point forward.

Even through her short stays in the hospital to have her trach tube changed, when she got her strength back, she would always go back to the Center for Living. She no longer had to go into the clinic to have her trach tube changed, as I was trained and am now responsible for changing the tube once a month. Since this point, we have been on a roll with the help of her doctors, therapists, and the exercise director at the Duke Center for Living.

Sometimes I feel that our roles as mother and daughter have changed because I am very strict with her, just as she was with me when I was a child. I don't allow her to eat certain things. I don't allow her to visit New Jersey as often as she would like, and I make sure she gets up on time and makes all of her appointments. My family members tease me, and they call me nurse Ratchet. I can sometimes feel the tension between my mother and me because I know she doesn't like this role reversal. She is a proud mother of six that still has all of her wits about her. We have our good days and our bad days (95% good), as we both understand that there has to be a balance. I'm willing do anything within my power, along with God's grace, to assist in keeping my mother alive and doing well.

Four years later, I remarried to a wonderful man who is very supportive of my caregiver role and all that it entails. Mom and I, along with God's grace, have been going strong for four years now with no hospital stays. We've been maintaining, vacationing and living a very fulfilled life, even with her trach and need for oxygen 24hrs a day. She was able to attend my wedding over in the Bahamas via cruise ship. We even went on a second cruise the following year and spent a few extra days hanging out in Miami. Mom hasn't missed a beat. I attribute that to her accepting her new lifestyle and making it work for her, instead of letting it hold her back. In the summer of 2007, after returning from one of her visits up to New Jersey, she had to be admitted back to Duke ICU where she was treated for fluid. While in New Jersey, she wasn't as active and the fluid had built up to a dangerous level. She had gained 15-20 lbs in two months and most of that was water weight. One thing I have learned is that one can never let up when one has a respiratory infection. The smallest thing can turn into something major. The lack of exercise for a month resulted in weight gain, which lead to the fluid gain, which also lead to an increased gas level in her blood. Through it all, God has blessed us with nearly five years of no hospital stays or major complications. I think this was His way getting her a well needed tune up. The doctors again brought up the need for mom to lose weight so that possibly the trach could be removed. The trach was intended only to be a temporary solution to a long term problem. The doctors even discussed weight loss surgery but feared her heart couldn't handle it.

After a one week stay, she was released and she was placed on a more strict diet. I took my mother home and we tried to pick up where we left off. I ended up having to leave for two weeks for a business trip to Canada so I left my two sisters in charge while I was gone. Four days after leaving for Canada, I got a phone call that my mother was back in the hospital. My initial response was to catch the next flight out of there and run to my mother's bedside. When caring for an elderly parent, support of other family members is good to have. My oldest sister told me to stay right where I was and that she and my other sister would look after our mother. Doing so was hard for me because it was I who drove mother to every doctor appointment. I was the one that spent nights sleeping in that uncomfortable chair while she was in the hospital.

Again, the decision was a hard one but I'm glad I stayed in Canada because doing so gave my sisters an opportunity to have that hands-on experience and be more involved in her care. She was hospitalized for the same thing, as she never fully recovered when she was released from the hospital a month prior. I was back in the United States in time to bring her home from the hospital, which was a blessing.

Since the hospital stay back in November, 2007, we've been maintaining, vacationing, and living a very fulfilled life. Now understanding more and more what the doctors meant when they said that there were gonna be some good days and some bad days. In January, 2010, my mother was admitted back in the hospital. This time was worse than all the others because I could see in my mother's eyes that she was tired. Her struggle had been going on for eight years now, and for the first time, she expressed to me that she had no desire to fight any longer. Each time, while on the ventilator, she would write down what she wanted to say. My family and I would make a game out of it and would laugh to no end but this time wasn't funny. Here I am, the only one at the hospital at the time, and she writes the words, "let die." I immediately rebuked those words and I stood on God's promise. I had to stand strong and firm in front of her, just as she did to me many times when I was a child, though I later fell apart. What became very apparent to me was that my mother was trying to fight this battle in her own strength, so I got to praying. People have the right to believe what they want to believe, but I believe in the power of prayer. We have to let go and let God fight our battles for us. From here to New Jersey, we were praying. I watched her strength and desire to live grow day by day, as God was working in the background. By now we know the drill. Get the fluid off and the blood gas level down so she can go back home. In time, she finally got down to a satisfactory level and away we went, only to go back to the hospital a month later. That time was because she was losing blood as a result of a change made to her medication. The anxiety from the procedure to check her blood level lead to her pressure going up and her blood gas level increasing, so, once again there were issues.

Almost a year has passed since we were released from Duke. I say, "we", because the group is my mother, Jesus, and me. Through it all, I have never left her side. I know that I am doing exactly what God had planned for my life. Mother may get around a little more slowly these days but she is still getting around. We celebrated her 75th birthday last year with all the family and what a celebration it was. The doctors no longer talk about her having to lose weight so they can remove the trach. She has learned to live with the trach and they have decided to leave well enough alone. She has been through so much and she has come a mighty long way. I think, with the continued love and support from family, friends, doctors, Duke Center for Living, and Jesus, she'll be with us for many more years to come. We are still maintaining, vacationing, and living a very fulfilled life.

I love you Mom.

# GIFTS OF THE JOURNEY

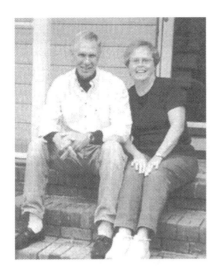

## *A Story of Discoveries Along the Path*

SHEER PANIC! Stomach sinking and heart racing, I listened, unable to concentrate, as the doctor explained my husband's diagnosis. "Your lungs have been damaged and you should be on oxygen twenty-four hours a day for the rest of your life. You are not going to get any better." She was forthright and abrupt. I just remember the shock of those words. How could this be? He was so young, only 58 years old.

My husband was being discharged from Buffalo General Hospital after suffering a pulmonary embolism in his right lung. I immediately panicked as I saw this as such a loss of freedom. We had watched his father suffer from lung disease and now I was fearful of what was to come. My feelings upon facing this diagnosis were apprehension and despair. I worried about what my husband must have been feeling and my own fear of the unknown. I felt anger, shock, and an inability to communicate what I was thinking. I did not want to upset him more. What was going to happen? How would he handle it? He always took care of everything. What would I do? I worried about his becoming depressed because he was always the strong one. He was the one I leaned on in times of trouble. We had just returned from Houston, Texas, and we were euphoric for the miracle the doctors felt considering the extent of his surgery and recovery. My husband had always been my rock and now I was afraid that my rock was crumbling.

That was eleven years ago, about a month after my husband had undergone surgery for a thoracic aortic aneurysm and an abdominal aneurysm at Methodist Hospital in Houston, Texas. He had been through so much. As we sat in the doctor's office that day in Buffalo and were told that my husband had a thoracic aortic aneurysm, my question was, "Can we schedule this as soon as possible? He will have eight weeks to recover. We have almost two months before the wedding."

Our youngest daughter had graduated from UNC Chapel Hill and was getting married on campus in a few months. The doctor looked at me in a rather forlorn way. "I don't think you realize the seriousness of this surgery," he said. In that instant my stomach sank. Now I cannot believe how naïve I was. I sure had to grow up in a hurry. I had never had to make the serious decisions in our life. My husband was always there for me. Trembling, my eyes began to fill with tears. I could not speak. After all, we had been told by a small town doctor that this was not very serious. The doctor suggested that we have some tests to see if the aneurysm had dissected and if not we should "go to North Carolina, see our daughter's wedding, and return immediately for surgery."

So we did what the doctor ordered, checked into the hospital, had all the tests run, and were given a clearance to go. There were a few conditions. "No Outer Banks for a vacation. No golf. Do not get into an accident. And return immediately after the wedding," were the doctor's words. He added, "I am not God. I can't predict what will happen but I think that is what you should do. The risks of surgery are high, and I think you should attend your daughter's wedding first."

So, away we went. We did not have time to worry. We traveled to North Carolina and continued the preparation for the wedding. Everything went along as planned. In a picturesque setting, amidst deep evergreens and magnificent blossoming magnolias of showy white flowers, the proud father escorted the elegant bride down the sculpturesque flagstone stairway.

The next Monday morning, we headed back to New York to meet with our doctor. As we walked into his office, he gave me a great big hug and said, "I did not want to ruin your daughter's wedding, but, Don, you have three aneurysms. Not only do you have a serious thoracic aortic aneurysm, you also have an abdominal and a femoral aneurysm. I would like you to go Methodist Hospital in Houston, Texas, to see Dr. Coselli who specializes in this type of surgery and has a reputation for having 'God gifted hands'."

After a whirlwind of phone calls and confirmations, we were on our way to Houston. Honeymoon destination changes for our daughter and new son-in-law quickly took place. Instead of Buffalo and Niagara Falls, they came to Houston.

As my husband and I boarded the plane that day I knew that I had to place myself in God's hands and rely on my faith to get us through. The time had come to slow down, face reality, pray, and meditate. The technique proved to be life-saving for my emotions.

Upon our arrival, our daughter and son-in-law surprised us at the airport. Their immediate presence reduced so much of the stress and anxiety of the unknown. We knew they were coming for the surgery but this took away all the worry and apprehension of being on our own. Unbeknownst to me, she had already researched all that she could at Washington University in St. Louis where she was working on her master's degree. She was prepared to ask questions that I could not even anticipate.

We were scheduled to see Dr. Coselli the next day. With butterflies and nerves aflutter, we entered the hospital. He was first announced by one of his staff. I felt a surge of panic as I realized the importance of the person I was about to meet. I had heard that people from all over the world came to him for treatment, which caused me to wonder how we were so blessed to be there. A member of his staff informed us that, "He had his own medical staff members assisting him and he asks them to follow specific protocols." Not all personnel were happy with his request for his own team, but they obliged.

He quickly dispelled our frayed nerves and put us at ease as he explained the procedure and answered our questions. He came right to the point. He told my husband that he was a picture of health and the only reason he was there was that he had been a smoker. Though the doctor was important and his expectations were high, he put us at ease with his reassuring and confident manner. After many questions, he replied to our daughter, "I am very impressed with your research." We were very proud.

Surgery took place two days later, and my husband did remarkably well. After many prayers and the expertise of this excellent team, doctors and nurses considered his case a miracle. He recovered in one of the shortest periods of time, with no paralysis and a wonderful prognosis. He was discharged from the hospital in five days. We stayed in Houston for a few weeks for follow-up appointments. Our flight home was uneventful, and he did very well the first week.

The next turn of events happened quickly. After a week, my husband developed some pain in his left leg and went to see the local doctor, who dismissed it as lack of exercise. Two days later, he was rushed to the hospital with a pulmonary embolism. After being transferred to Buffalo General Hospital, the doctors again considered his survival a miracle.

But, then we were told that his lungs were damaged and that he would have to be on oxygen for the remainder of his life. We thought he was doing so well that he would eventually resume normal activities. As we sat there that morning, I remember the sinking feeling I had as I looked at my husband's face and knew that he was not accepting this diagnosis very well. After all, he had never been sick, was an avid golfer, traveled around the world, a perfect picture of health before all of this happened. He had just taken an early retirement. We were about to travel and enjoy life. The experience seemed surreal. How could this be happening? Where were we headed? What was he thinking and feeling? Was he as scared as I was? Could I handle anymore? I know that God only gives us what we can handle, but hadn't we already handled enough? I felt that we had done so well coping with the initial diagnosis, plus he survived. What was next? I had to stay strong for him, but I was scared. Apparently the combination of the surgery and pulmonary embolism presented another hurdle to overcome.

No one knows how he or she will react when confronted with terrifying news. I had no idea of the inner strength I possessed and developed when I relied on my faith. My faith was always important to me and I had considered myself blessed to be where I was on that part of my spiritual journey yet I never realized the power of that belief. All I know is that I never prayed so hard during this time, and I never felt so strong in all of my life. I have read that God is always with us in our darkest of hours but now I know that He is! I also learned that all of our life's experiences are only preparation for the next step. We may begin with baby steps but we eventually are able to take giant strides.

Following my husband's recovery, we decided to relocate from New York to North Carolina. While our daughter was attending UNC Chapel Hill, we had fallen in love with the area. She was now married, living in Durham, and working at Duke Hospital.

She especially wanted us to make the move so that her father could be close to some of the best doctors in the country.

Upon relocating, our first mission was to establish a relationship with one of the best pulmonologists possible. Our daughter recommended Dr. K, and my husband was fortunate to get an appointment within a short time. After running many tests, Dr. K's first recommendation was to join the Duke Center for Living Campus Pulmonary Program for pre and post-operative lung transplant patients. Because my husband was not a transplant patient, we had no idea what to expect. The first meeting was a little unnerving as we listened to everyone's story. However, we quickly realized that, while all the stories were different, everyone experienced the same fear and apprehension. The program helped us both so much. As we listened to everyone's story, we forgot about our own and became a unit of people caring for one other.

Coming to terms with what was to happen took some time, not to mention our concern becoming one of getting in the best shape possible to handle whatever came our way. We needed to develop the discipline and determination that we saw in the patients we met. I knew that a healthy diet and exercise were the best way to get my husband in good physical shape. Little did I know the benefits that we would both derive from this program. They far exceeded anything I could imagine. The physical benefits are apparent, but I was clueless as to the psychological, emotional, and spiritual aspects. The constant attention, the insight, the kindness and dedication extended by the staff to their patients is a very moving sight and is evidenced in each one's courage and endurance each day. That there is a reason we cross paths with others is easy to see. The growth in mind, body, and spirit is undeniable. This has taken me to a whole new place of discovery.

I am still exercising today at the Center after joining the spousal program more than five years ago. When offered the opportunity to join, I jumped at the chance. I knew I needed to get into an exercise routine and develop some self-discipline. I also felt it would be encouraging for my husband to have me exercising along with him. I cannot begin to explain all that this program has taught me, but I do know that I learned a lot about life. The people I have met, their spirit, their strength, their will to live, along with their kindness and willingness to share their stories, have taught me more about life than life itself. Living life to the fullest and being there for others is the most powerful prescription there is.

Yes, I was scared when I came here . . . riddled with anxiety, afraid of the unknown, fearing the worst. But what I have gained is immeasurable, and my husband's perspective on the future has changed. He has found out that he is not alone and that life offers many opportunities if one just partakes of what is offered. I have learned that we are in the place that we are supposed to be at this time of our lives for a reason while our learning curves continue.

*Lorraine Williamson*

# WHY I CHOSE A PROFESSION IN RESPIRATORY THERAPY

# Seeing a Patient as a Person

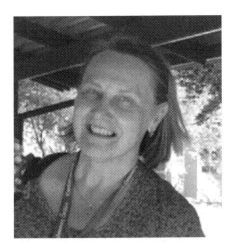

## *A Story from a Therapists View*

"What do you want to be when you grow up?" "Nurse", was my first response. The years passed and I spent most of my time participating in team sports, gymnastics, baton corps and dance. This led to the girl athlete award of my senior class which sent me onward to Slippery Rock State University for a double major in Health and Physical Education. Gone were the thoughts of Nursing . . . teaching was the dream . . .

Years later . . . major crossroads . . . I went back to school for respiratory therapy. I wondered how the time, effort, and cost of two seemingly different vocations could be interrelated if at all.

Then God took the multiple pieces of my life and created a quilt. The pattern formed Pulmonary Rehabilitation. A therapist stopped me one day and asked if I had a degree and I answered yes, in Education. My major was Health and Physical Education.

His response was "wow, you'd be great for pulmonary rehab. We'll talk about it!"

My career in pulmonary rehab spans almost twenty years. I consider myself a pulmonary rehab specialist (my own title). I've worked in three different hospitals, participated in a Lung Volume Reduction Study, provided satellite programs for lung transplant patients in the Philadelphia area and I'm now working in one of the most well-known intensive pulmonary rehab programs in the US.

What exactly is my role as a Respiratory Therapist specializing in Pulmonary Rehabilitation?

I guide and encourage each patient under my care successfully through a physical exercise program and education. Sound easy? Have you ever had your wind knocked out or choked on something until you lost your breath? Can you ride a bike breathing through a straw? Try it. Individuals with chronic lung disease are starving for air. Getting out of a chair, walking in their homes, even sitting and eating dinner can completely wipe them out!!

Imagine the expressions and comments I hear when I tell them this program is one month, five days a week, three to four hours a visit and will involve walking, biking, floor exercise and weight lifting! These same individuals (who think I must be crazy, but don't have a better alternative) generally thrive in rehab. They gain strength, confidence and understanding of their disease. They learn to cope with chronic illness and discover what care and treatment options are available. They meet people with similar problems and needs. They make friends and build support systems.

# What do I contribute?

A watchful eye to keep them safe, a helping hand when needed, the knack of knowing when to say, "stay a little longer" or "stop, you've had enough". Ears to listen. The knowledge to teach and the courage to stay the course with each one of these wonderful people.

*Carol Carson*

BS, RCP

# WHEN TRANSPLANT IS THE SOLUTION

# My Second Chance

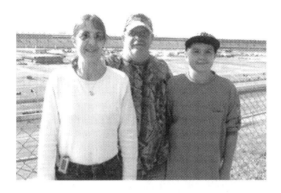

## *A Story of Determination*

Hi. My name is Crystal Akins. I am a 48-year-old mother with Cystic Fibrosis, and I've had a double lung transplant. Growing up, I was reasonably healthy, dealing only with Bronchitis or Pneumonia. I was 19 the first time I was hospitalized with a need for IV antibiotics. For a few years, I was in and out of the hospital often.

Each stay was for at least two weeks. During that time I discovered that I had Pseudomonas, a bacteria that lives in the lungs. Over the years, I had many infections and hospital stays. In my mid-thirties, I met and married my husband. I had a very healthy pregnancy, despite the risks. Also, I am a diabetic. As our son began to get older, I noticed a gradual decline of my lung functions.

In September, 2006, my pulmonologist convinced me to go to Boston to learn about lung transplantation. At that point

I was not on oxygen and wasn't convinced I wanted or needed a transplant. The statistics of success rate and survival rate did nothing to encourage me. At the same time, my brother who also has Cystic Fibrosis, started pursuing a lung transplant in Pennsylvania. He was on oxygen and was finding it limiting. He went back and forth for a couple of years before going to Florida to try another hospital. They referred him to Duke University, in North Carolina, late in 2008. He had a successful transplant in May, 2009.

In March, 2009, I was hospitalized for a pseudomonas, MRSA, and serratia infection. When I was discharged, I went home on oxygen. Prior to that, I'd always gotten rid of the oxygen before leaving the hospital. I was still naïve and believed my O2 would get better. My doctor told me that I was retaining CO2. I started needing IV antibiotics about every two months for flare ups. When my brother came home in August, 2009, he told me to contact Duke University. He did not want me to allow myself to get as sick as he had become.

I went to Duke University for an evaluation the first week of November, 2009. The doctors felt I had potential to be a candidate and asked me to come back as soon as possible. They told me that I would need to gain weight and suggested a feeding tube. They also wanted me to enroll in their rehab program to build up my strength. My husband and I flew back to N.Y. Unfortunately, no one had told me that flying with diminished lung capacity is a bad idea. On the flight, while using portable oxygen, my O2 level fell to 77. That night I went to the emergency room because I was still having difficulty breathing. The E.R. staff gave me some fluids for dehydration, along with oxygen, and then sent me home. The following day I was taken back to the hospital and admitted. I had another severe infection, and my CO2 (carbon dioxide) levels were climbing. I was there five days, worsening each day.

On November 12, 2009, I was flown back to Duke University, on a medical flight, to be treated. At that point, I weighed 89 pounds and had to walk with a walker because I had no muscle strength. I stayed there for thirteen days. During that time, I had a feeding tube implanted. I also had physical therapy. I was discharged the day before Thanksgiving and no longer needed a walker. The following Monday, I started my rehab at The Center for Living, which consisted of one hour of floor exercises, 20-30 minutes of walking, and 20 minutes of weights. In three weeks, I gained ten pounds. On December 16, 2009, I was officially listed on the National Transplant List. Two days later, I got my first call that the doctors had possibly found a set of lungs. This ended up being my first dry run. I also had dry runs on December 24th, 27th, 28th, and, again, on January 3, 2010.

Then on January 7, 2010, I got the official "it's a go" and got my lungs. The following day I was taken off the ventilator and was encouraged to walk. I was moved out of ICU the following evening and continued to walk. On January 11, 2010, my heart stopped. I was revived and taken back to ICU and placed back on the ventilator. The next day I was stable enough to again be taken off the ventilator. The day after that I was again moved from ICU to begin my in-hospital rehabilitation.

On January 19, 2010, I was released from the hospital to begin my outpatient rehabilitation at The Center for Living. Before my surgery, I had gotten up to 114 pounds. When I was discharged, I was back down to 90 pounds. I was allowed to drink only thickened liquids with my medicines and tube feed. The doctors did not want me to aspirate into my new lungs. On February 7, 2010, I had to have my feeding tube replaced because it had turned upon itself. I was in the hospital for four days. On February 26, 2010, I had a Toupet procedure done, a partial stomach wrap. Then I was allowed nothing by mouth for two weeks to allow the swelling to go down. In the middle of March, I started on clear liquids for one week. I was then allowed soft, solid food, which landed me back in the hospital because my inflammation had not gone down, and some food material was stuck in my esophagus. I had to have the waste pumped and was allowed nothing by mouth for another month. I spent another four days in the hospital. The last week of March, I passed my swallow test and was again allowed to have clear liquids.

One week later, I was told I could start on a full liquid diet. I was also told I was healthy and strong enough to return to N.Y. This was a happy day even though I would need to return to Duke in three weeks for a check-up and a bronchoscopy. On February 2, 2010, I had had a mild rejection, which was treated with solumedrol and step down of prednisone for 12 days. Then on March 23rd, I had another mild rejection, which, again, was treated again with solumedrol and step down of prednisone. On May 4, 2010, I had my feeding tube removed and the following day I had another bronchoscopy that showed another mild rejection. This time I had to be admitted to the hospital for a RAT-G treatment. This is a three day treatment. I was back to Duke on June 22, 2010, for another bronchoscopy from which I got a clean bill of health (No rejection). I was back again on August 3, 2010, and my bronchoscopy showed no rejection. I have to return on October 25th and am hoping for more of the same. After I returned home, there was a readjustment period. Of course, there were the daily exercises and slowly incorporating the household routine and errands. My family and friends were happy to have me home and amazed at the change. We started walking one mile every day. Before walking outside was too cold, I had gotten up to two and a half miles a day. During the summer, I took up kayaking and would swim laps when I got the chance. I plan on snowshoeing this winter.

One important thing I learned was to never stop moving. One has to keep pushing one's self in order to stay as strong as possible. Remember, exercise is the best medicine and rehab programs are wonderful.

*Crystal M. Akins*

# My Pulmonary Journey

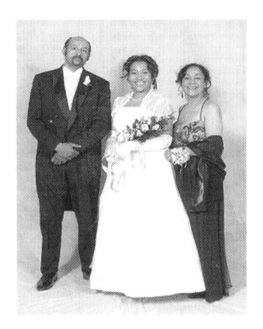

## *A Story of Living Life with New Lungs*

I was diagnosed with Sarcoidosis (a disease of unknown cause, characterized by granulomatous tubercles of the skin, lymph nodes, lungs, eyes and other organs) approximately twenty-two years ago, following the birth of my daughter. I experienced some shortness of breath and tightness in the chest. My sister, a family practitioner, suggested that I get an x-ray of my chest. It showed some spotting on the lungs. She ordered a bronchoscopy, an examination by means of a bronchoscope. A bronchoscope is a lighted, flexible tubular instrument that is inserted into the trachea for diagnosis and for removing inhaled objects. This indicated that I did have Sarcoidosis.

During that time, I had check-ups such as chest x-rays, pulmonary function tests, and blood work. However, a period of time went by in which my breathing worsened. I started to get granuloma on the skin, especially on the ears, around the nose, and on the scalp. My pulmonologist referred me to a dermatologist who administered steroidal injections on those areas regularly. The steroidal injections kept my granuloma at bay only temporarily. The steroidal injections were necessary every month. Because of the injections, my scalp was so tender that it would actually bleed.

The shortness of breath was beginning to be a problem at work. I was employed by the Centers for Disease Control and Prevention in Atlanta, Georgia, as an Employee Development Specialist and Conference Planner. I remember having difficulty walking up and down stairs. Also, when I had to give presentations, I would have difficulty breathing and talking at the same time. I never will forget mornings getting ready for work. I would lay my clothes out at night so I could move more efficiently to get ready in the morning. I had to stop wearing perfume because shortness of breath would occur, and I would feel light headed. It was one afternoon that I was arriving to my mother's house to pick up my daughter, that, as I walked in the door, I actually almost fell to the floor. Luckily, my father and brother were there to break the fall.

My pulmonologist discussed placing me in a pulmonary program at the hospital and the use of oxygen therapy for my lungs. I walked short distances on a track and lifted weights. The program was every day except Saturday and Sunday. I was on two units of oxygen twenty-four hours a day, seven days a week. Walking down the hospital corridor became harder and harder for me until, eventually, I had to use a wheelchair. Results of my pulmonary function tests continued to worsen.

Our house was three stories. However, I could only stay on the main floor. My job gave me permission to work from home. Working from home helped a great deal because there were times that I drove into work and was so lightheaded that I had to wait at least five minutes to go into my office.

One morning my husband and I awoke to my having a horrific breathing episode. He had me breathe into a brown paper bag because I was hyperventilating. He called an ambulance right away. The emergency rescue man had to carry me out to the ambulance. I was unable to walk by myself. I thought my lung had collapsed. We rushed to the hospital. I lay on the stretcher, still unable to catch my breath. I prayed so hard to God that I was not dying. The experience was so frightening. I thought I was going to pass out. The emergency doctors put me on a morphine drip. Everything started to calm down; however, things in the room looked dark to me. Needless to say, I had an adverse reaction to a drug. A few hours later I was feeling a little bit better. The family was talking about having me airlifted to Duke University Medical Center in Durham, North Carolina. There was not a life flight available from the hospital on the weekend. That night, I was admitted to the hospital. My family had spent a great deal of time researching Duke as a place for further pulmonary care. The data showed that it had a great success rate for lung transplantations.

While I was in the hospital, the doctors took more tests. They had a lung transplantation program; however, it was not up to Duke's standards. The doctors suggested a lung transplant. At this point, I was end stage Sarcoidosis/pulmonary hypertension.

My family and I headed to Durham, North Carolina, in July, 2004. Before we met with the Duke doctors, we wanted to seek a second opinion. We met with the best Sarcoidosis specialist in the area, a Dr. Donohue at the University of North Carolina, Chapel Hill, Hospital. Unfortunately for me, he listened to my lungs and told me clearly that the time had come for a lung transplant. That was my only option.

We met (I in a wheelchair) with the Duke transplant team doctors. I had to take various tests to ensure I would be a good candidate for a lung transplant. My tests came back that I would be a good candidate. I was introduced to the Duke Fitness Center, or, Center for Living. The pulmonary therapists were wonderful and very knowledgeable. The program consisted of floor exercises, walking the track, and cybex weight lifting. My starting the program prior to surgery was imperative. My mother stayed with me and joined the Center for Living. She was getting her exercise as well.

I was listed on the United Network for Organ Sharing in September. I thanked God so very much for making this possible. I was so anxious to move on with my life. My mother was going back to Atlanta early October, the same month my husband arrived. We made arrangements for my daughter to stay in Atlanta with my sister and dad so that she could finish her semester as a high school junior.

My prayers were answered. I remember "the call" that I received from my transplant coordinator that I must get to the hospital immediately! James and I were so nervous. I actually asked the transplant coordinator if I could take a shower.

The wait seemed hours. We thought that maybe my new lungs were somewhere in the hospital. The time must have been around 11:00 p.m., October 30th. James said that I was very calm before I went into the operating room. I did not feel nervous or afraid anymore. I had a one-on-one with God. I asked him to stay with me. I felt him by my side. My surgery was approximately eleven hours. The surgeon told James that my bad lungs were like concrete.

After the surgery, I experienced a great deal of air-way constriction. My loving husband had to take me to the hospital a number of times for this breathing issue as well as post-surgical infections that I had developed. I cannot recall the number of bronchoscopies and hospitalizations I had. My air-way would be cut off because of the plugs (mucous) that would not come out by themselves. I eventually had two stents placed on my bronchus to alleviate the problem. I was also on nebulizer treatments. I experienced severe, chronic pain in my chest. It was so severe I sometimes cried. While in the hospital, my own doctor came in to see me. I pleaded with him to help me. I could not stop crying. The pain doctors came to see me. They administered two drugs that I still take for the pain, oxycontin® and lyrica®. James and I decided to make Durham our home, the best choice for us since I was having so many complications.

I continue to control my chronic pain to this day, even though my surgery was seven years ago. I also continue to exercise at the Center for Living. My husband has been my rock through it all. He is with me every step of the way. He has spent endless nights staying awake to watch me. He is wonderful to still keep up with all my medications. I could not have made this pulmonary journey without him. Thanks to God for having given me a second chance in life. I will live it to the fullest!

*Edwina Stratton*

# Random Acts of Kindness and Thanksgiving

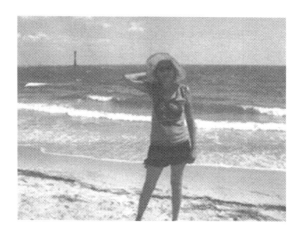

## *A Story of Gratitude*

I am grateful to have been practicing and experiencing random acts of kindness for many years now. I truly believe that sweet acts of selflessness are what connect us as we travel this sometimes difficult journey called life.

On July 15, 2010, I experienced the greatest act of selfless giving possible. I received the gift of new life through a double lung transplant. The gift of these lungs has changed everything in my world. I am talking without gasping for breath, sleeping through the night without waking up winded. I am blessed beyond measure to be able to actually walk on Folly Beach, kick my feet up in the chilly surf, drag my toes through the cool, moist sand and get back to my car, all without use of an oxygen tank and without being so worn out that I couldn't drive myself home.

Many of us take simple day-to-day tasks quite for granted, but when you're 43 years old and told that you can no longer work and must live on supplemental oxygen 24/7; you don't take very much for granted at all. I missed doing all the fun things in life, like traveling, socializing and walking on the beach. I also missed the simpler things, like being able to clean my own home, go to the movies or even be part of the important relationships in my life.

I don't know anything about the person whose life was lost or about the family and friends who grieved, who are likely still grieving that life, but I know that that person's gift of organ donation has given me a new life. I'm busy living as many moments of it as I possibly can. I don't want to take for granted one more moment, one more person, or one more chance to be a part of this beautiful journey. I intend to honor the lovely soul who thought to sign an organ donor card by living this new life as fully and as happily as ever as possible!

# My Christmas Miracle

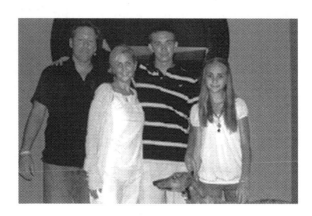

## *A Story of Receiving One of Life's Greatest Gifts*

On a bleak January night in 2006, as I was sitting on my stiff and uncomfortable hospital bed, I was given devastating news. I was told that I was dying because my lungs were failing, and that I needed a double lung transplant in order to survive.

I have Cystic Fibrosis (CF), a genetic disease that can damage the respiratory system, digestive tract, and reproductive system. I was a very healthy child and never had any illnesses to speak of, but, I mysteriously began getting chronic lung infections in high school. The doctors had a hard time diagnosing me because I mainly displayed problems with my respiratory system. After years of testing different medications and visiting new doctors, my illness was eventually labeled as a variant of CF. As a teenager who just wanted to fit in, being ill was hard to accept. I became rebellious and didn't want anyone to know that I had the illness. I just wanted to be treated like a normal person. Relying on my parents, I counted on them to get me the treatments and care I needed. I tried to hide my illness from others as much as possible. After I married, I depended on my husband for help. Being an amazing caregiver, he became my parent in many ways while helping me deal with countless infections and hospitalizations. We struggled together through many rough days, yet, I always seemed to bounce back.

I was 37 years old when I was told the news that I needed a lung transplant. My doctors came into my hospital room and were not gentle in their approach. After they left, I felt as though I had been given a death sentence. I went through all the stages of dealing with death. I couldn't believe this was happening to me. Would I actually get a transplant? I loved my lungs; they were, after all, mine. For a few days after I was discharged from the hospital, I couldn't think straight. I thought that maybe I would be okay and that I didn't really need a transplant. Yet, I was very sick and needed to accept the reality of it all. I knew that this time in the hospital was different because I was put on oxygen and had to go home with an oxygen tank. I was told that, with only 15% lung function, I would need to be connected to oxygen for the rest of my life, or until after transplant, *if* I decided to have surgery. Being on oxygen was a very hard thing to get used to. I knew that I couldn't accept it. I was very self-conscious in public and had to get used to stares and even questions from strangers about why I needed oxygen. The time had come to decide . . . did I want to live or die? The answer was obvious. I was going to fight like hell to live. Looking at my two beautiful children and loving husband, I thought about the wonderful future I could look forward to with them. I hated the idea of my missing out on so much of our lives. The next eleven months were spent going through series after series of tests and preparations in order to be put on the lung transplant list. The ironic thing about being placed on the transplant list is that you have to be sick enough to need the lungs but healthy enough to survive the surgery. Being sick enough was easy. Getting in shape for the surgery was another difficult passage.

Physically preparing for such an intensive and invasive procedure was, at times excruciating, but also unbelievably empowering. My body and mind were tested in ways I never thought possible. I had to be strong emotionally and physically. Despite the doctor's grim outlook and the fact that they gave me only a few weeks to live before I was activated in December of 2006, I knew that I had to believe in myself. I knew that my outlook played a huge part in my survival as much as my body. In order to survive and heal, my spirituality, my positive attitude, my will, and my desire to live had to be very strong. Eventually, I made peace with the idea of getting new lungs and was actually excited for surgery. My husband and children were anticipating the surgery, too. My husband would get his wife back and my children could get their mommy back. Many remarkable things happened during the eleven months waiting to be activated. I grew more in those eleven months than I had in my previous years. I took nothing for granted. I began to cherish the beauty around me in nature and in simple things. During a month long stay in the hospital just before transplant, my husband wheeled me outside for some fresh air. Almost four weeks had passed since I had seen the sun. My hospital room window faced a wall. Finally, being able to be outside even for only a short time, I felt a new awareness that may only come to those who experience a life-changing event. It was October and the leaves were gently falling to the ground while the sun filtered through the trees. The breathtaking scene reminded me of a Monet painting. I experienced the most amazing feeling as the sun hit my face. It was as though a miracle was happening right then. Tears rolled down my face, and I smiled at my husband. We both knew how significant that moment was. I wondered how all the other people around seemed to miss it. Were they too busy to notice the splendor of the scene? I wondered why I didn't see it until now, the beauty all around me. Before my transplant, I was in the hospital for over a month and lost 20 precious pounds. I felt defeated. Just to sit up, was a struggle, but I really wanted to live, thrive, and prove to the doctors that I could do it just like I did when I delivered two beautiful, healthy babies years before. I knew in my heart that I could survive surgery and live a full life. I imagined myself on a beach without an oxygen (O2) tank, running, laughing and breathing, with my new, healthy lungs. I couldn't wait to start my second life with them. I did find myself worrying about the donor, though. Someone would have to die for me to live. That fact was hard to accept. I came to realize, though, that the person would not die because of me, he or she would die even without me. Yet, I would live because of the individual. The donor was caring enough to think of someone else by becoming an organ donor. I felt that it was my responsibility to try to live my life to its fullest in appreciation of him or her.

On December 23rd 2006, I finally got THE CALL!! It was nine days after I was activated! All I could think about was the donor and his or her family. I cried, said a prayer, and tried to regain composure as we headed to the hospital. I called my brother, my parents, and a few close friends after the nurse told me that the lungs were a perfect fit for me. I remember looking at my husband and thinking what a miracle this all was. My children joined me in my bed as I was wheeled down to surgery. It was a ride of a lifetime. I was so happy and proud of myself for being able to get to that point.

The very next morning I was walking the hospital intensive care unit (ICU) halls with chest tubes, catheters, and several IV's, but NO oxygen tank!! I was ecstatic! Nine days later I was out of the hospital and back to rehab where I was to spend several weeks gaining strength to start my new life. I surprised everyone except my husband and kids with my swift recovery. I was so excited to start living again that I could barely contain myself. I felt so fortunate that things went so smoothly. Preparation and patience were keys to my recovery. Before and after surgery, I tried to stay out of bed, even if it just meant sitting upright in a chair. I tried to walk as much as possible on the clinic treadmill, eat healthy and follow doctor's orders. Planning fun and exciting things to do in the future also had a huge impact on how I handled the transplant experience.

It has been almost four years now since my transplant and I feel so blessed. LIFE is amazing. I look at it as an opportunity to experience new things, spend time with those I love, and also share my story, both with those who are sick and those who are well. I hope my story inspires people to see the good in LIFE and not focus on the bad. The mind is a powerful tool. Believing in yourself can change your life! I see every day as a gift and I am forever thankful to my donor for giving me a second chance. What a miracle it is!

The best gift one can give is the gift of life.

*Kristina Kelso*

# The Pink Elephant in My Life

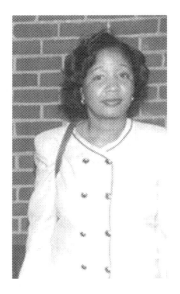

*A Story of One Woman's 40Year Battle with*
*Sarcoidosis*

I will always remember that October day when my pulmonary doctor called me to come to his office. He asked if my husband could meet us. I knew immediately that this was not good news. The doctor informed me that I had developed secondary hypertension. I didn't know what to do. He told me there was no cure for pulmonary hypertension. I thought about going to my pastor but immediately decided against it. Should I call my mom? Why bother her with this? I got into my car and drove. My husband and children were not at home, so I just cried, screamed, and cried more until no more tears would come. The thought of going onto perpetual oxygen was unacceptable to me. Little did I know that my journey was just beginning.

My journey started in 1973 when I was diagnosed with sarcoidosis. I had never heard of this disease before. I graduated with my Master's Degree from the University of Michigan, married, and landed my first job, all in 1972. I was feeling good emotionally and physically. Out of the blue, I began to feel tired, extremely tired. I lost weight without trying, and I developed this cough that became worse each day. Finally, I went to the family physician. He felt I was just having difficulty dealing with the stress of my husband's job. I told him that this was not the case. He prescribed Valium 5mg, b.i.d.

About a week later, I was awakened by pain on my left side. My husband drove me to the emergency room. The x-ray technicians took chest X-rays and decided to admit me because the doctor saw a spot on my lung. Following a two week hospitalization, I was diagnosed with sarcoidosis after experiencing a collapsed lung and having a liver biopsy. The doctor told me that, in 94% of the cases of sarcoidosis, the illness disappears. He told me I had a chronic condition, but to nurse it

Yet here I was 20 years later, crying over the idea of going on oxygen. I refused to wear the nasal cannula to work or out socially. For the next ten years, I managed somehow. I worked full time and constantly made excuses for the cough and my inability to walk up steps. Going to a conference at Yale nearly killed me as I had to walk everywhere that day. I think my coworkers felt I was lazy. The truth was that I was trying to breathe.

In 2000 I, with my husband, son, daughter, grandchild, and friend went to Boston for the christening of my granddaughter. On the way back (I didn't take my oxygen), I couldn't get air and asked to be taken to the nearest emergency room. I remember going to the front desk and just saying I needed oxygen. That was all I remember, and then everything went dark. God really took care of me because there was a doctor coming down the hallway of the emergency room. This doctor had seen this type of reaction before. He saved my life. I spent the night in intensive care. My daughter had to sleep in the hallway that night as she could not stay with me in intensive care.

This episode happened in January. I didn't make it back to work until the end of October. Staying at home was new for me. I would watch Jerry Springer, which helped me nap. I was just so weak. An intervention by my doctor at the University of Connecticut finally got me to use oxygen 24/7. I was referred to Dr. F. at Boston University. This guy was excellent. He told me that he was the last stop before transplantation. He explained Flolan® to me. I thought I understood what he was saying but I did not realize the responsibility that came with this medication. I had to mix medications every day and, when going out, I had to take a supply. I could not be disconnected from this medication.

Going back to work in October was one of the hardest things I have ever had to do in my life. I could tell right away that people did not treat me the same. Some just could not get over the weight loss. The people who were mean to me were the doctors. I remember my Department Chairman referring to me as a clown. Mean, too, was the resident who stated one must be in need of money or be very committed to working with his or her patients if one is working with that oxygen. What kept me going was the fact that Dr. "M". and Dr. "F". were very proud and encouraging of my working. I must admit that I also had been educated about my illness and realized that I had to plan for my future. I wanted my retirement and my insurance. I knew that God's grace and mercy would bring me to the point of retirement.

The doctor finally had the talk with me and my husband. He told us that I needed a transplant. Dr. "M" had already warned me that I might need a transplant some day. He would say the doctors like you to walk in as this increase your chances of walking out. Dr. "M" was pushing Chapel Hill. Dr. "F" was pushing Duke, having graduated from Duke. We reviewed the track records of both hospitals thoroughly. I went with Duke.

I retired on July 25, 2000. Rather, I went out on vacation time and sick time and, finally, was officially retired December 1, 2000. I arrived at the Center for Living in August, 2000. I lived with my mother about 20 minutes away. My mom was 83 and I felt good that I could still cook for her. My sister still gave my mother her bath, but I was still able to help. She always cooked a good meal for us every Sunday. When I went to church, I would drive alone in case I ran out of oxygen and needed to leave early.

Waiting for my transplant was hard. Sometimes, I would get very lonely for home. I missed my family and friends. At one point, I thought the transplant team had forgotten about me. I had to take a three week break before working on this story again. My emotions seemed to be going wild and I kept remembering good and bad things that happened to me while I was sick. When I felt that the transplant team had forgotten about me, things just started to happen. I remember coming home on a Thursday and feeling very tired. My mother told me not to cook because she was treating us. She gave me $20.00 to buy carry out. The telephone rang, and it was a call from Duke. The doctors had a lung for me. I called my sister Rosella to drive me and my other sister, Agrow, to get the word around that I had been called. I know my sister drove about 90 miles per hour. I told her she would kill us before we made it to the hospital. This was my second run. The first time was what we call a dry run.

My first run was cancelled but I got the pre-operative experience (All the blood work, x-rays, and a shower). I then got the call that the organ was not good. I was somewhat sad and relieved. The real thing was unbelievable. My family arrived and we prayed in my room. I was wheeled down the hall. I remember talking to two technicians about that with which they were going to sedate me. I awoke with tubes and a breathing machine. The picture did not look good for me. I remember seeing my friend, sister, husband, and nieces. I understood what was going on because we had been educated and I, in turn, had tried to prepare my family for what was to come.

I awoke with my husband standing by giving me comfort. He had been in Connecticut and I wondered how he got to North Carolina so soon. The rest is a blur. I do remember my friend coming back from Atlanta. The doctors told my family that I had a 50/50 chance of living. I remember that I could not speak and my hands were tied down. Then I knew how restraint feels. The nurses were afraid I would pull my tubes out in my sleep. I have spoken with several lung transplant patients about what they felt after surgery. One patient shared that he had nightmares while another patient shared that he kept stepping down into nothing. I had the dream of my life. To begin with, I was with Jesus and he took me on a tour of heaven. There were many mansions. There was also an island where people went who were not ready for heaven. When fit, they could cross the river into heaven. I saw another rehab patient who was with Jesus while I was on my tour. There were beautiful, vibrant flowers of purple, yellow, and white. Every building was made of gold.

There were also crazy things that I thought about also. I dreamed that my niece had given me Flolan® while I was in the hospital. The computer in which she gave me the Flolan® had infected other patients. We had to be moved to a Chinese restaurant: I could actually smell the food. I also thought that my brother's wife had been in a car accident and died. I was shocked when she showed up to visit me. How could this be? In short, those days after transplant were very hard. When the Thanksgiving holiday arrived, I couldn't eat, talk or write. I felt very weak. I was so hot and thirsty but my faith kept me going. I closed my eyes and God gave me holy water. He blew the Holy Spirit on me and I felt cool (what a wonderful feeling). Some people may not believe me but I was touched by God and this was due to prayers, my family, friends, and the church.

I just remember that there were tubes everywhere. There were tubes in my sides that drained fluid and air from the space around my lungs. I also had a catheter to drain urine output. A pulseoximeter was on my finger to measure or monitor pulse rate and oxygen levels in my blood. A large IV catheter was in the side of my neck and a tube in my mouth that was connected to a ventilator. In other words, the room was packed with machines. I had prepared my family but this was still hard.

The hardest thing I had to do was to come off of the breathing machine. I was afraid . . . very afraid. I remember the doctors started me off spending 15 minute intervals off the ventilator, et cetera. I watched the clock the whole time and, when my time was nearly up, I would call the nurse. That I could not breathe on my own was very hard for me to accept. God blessed me with the best transplant nurse in the whole, wide world—Jean. She gave me hope because she could reason with me. There was also the "Blonde Squad", as I called them, because they were young and blonde, worked well together, and they were determined that I would live (I still thank them to this day).

I came off the breathing machine and on December 23, 2002. I was discharged from the hospital. My discharge was difficult. My transplant nurse did her part but the residents made things rough for me. The list of medications was overwhelming. Prograf® at 10 and 10, Prednisone 20 daily, Protonix 50, Vitamins, et cetera. To my surprise, I also had to give myself shots of insulin. The manual I received before transplant indicated that some patients have to take insulin but I didn't realize I would be one.

On December 24, 2002, I had an appointment at the Center for Living. My family flew in that morning and came with me to that appointment. Thank God I was able to spend Christmas Eve with my family. I felt guilty because I did not have a Christmas tree, so I sent my husband to buy lights and we lit a plant. I could not cook so my husband prepared ribs.

Christmas Eve at the McCain's is usually a big deal. We went to my mother's house for Christmas. We arrived early to beat the crowd. My 83-year-old mother just sat in a corner in her favorite chair. She appeared to be overwhelmed. She was happy yet unable to express her feelings of joy. My family returned to Connecticut later that evening. I missed them but decided to put my energy into getting better. December 26, I was back in rehab with David pushing, showing no mercy as he probably felt I could do more.

The roles in my marriage were completely reversed. My husband shopped, cooked, washed the clothes, and, in general, took care of me. I made sure that my husband had time for himself. I encouraged him to work out at the gym where we lived. Having an outlet is important for caregivers. The support of my family and friend can never be overstated. My sister stayed with me after my husband left on New Year's Day. The following morning, my friend, Mattie, arrived and spent the week caring for me while a visiting nurse was also coming in every day. After Mattie left, I was alone. There were times when I was so lonely. My oldest sister would call and give me encouragement. Sleeping at night was difficult for me as I was always afraid someone would break in. Once I was able to drive, I felt a sense of independence, even if I could only drive to the center and hospital. Soon, however, I was driving on the interstate.

## A PRAYER FOR HEALING

God in heaven, I come as humble as I know how thanking you for all that you have done for me and will do for me in the future. God, you are the creator of the universe. You have the power to make all things happen. If we believe with the faith of a mustard seed, you said all things are possible. God, I ask in the name of your son, Jesus Christ, for healing. I repent of my sins and believe that you will heal me. I praise your holy name. These and other blessings I ask in name of your mighty son, Jesus Christ. Amen and Amen

Eight years have passed since my transplant. The road hasn't always been smooth but the journey has been worthwhile. I have had six hospitalizations since my transplant. The last one was for four days, February 6, 2007. One of the most important things that I remember is the smile from Dr. Davis one Saturday morning. That smile told me that I was going to be all right. It meant so much to me. I thank everyone for his or her love and support.

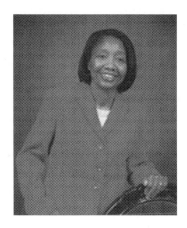

*Mary Crisp McClain*

# I've Been Blessed

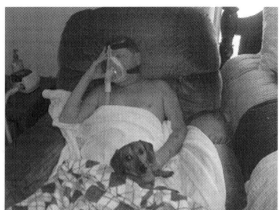

*A story of a man thankful to be alive*

There is nothing special about me. I'm just a regular 59-year-old man who was given the supreme gift in life—another chance. I have no idea why I was chosen for this second chance but I intend to do whatever I can to help whomever I can in all ways possible.

I was a long-time smoker who came from a family where many relatives had died from cancer, including my mother. I knew smoking was killing me but liked it so much I was willing to take the risk. I always thought I could not live without a cigarette when, in fact, the opposite was true. My health had been great my entire life, except for getting bronchitis every year. I had never been sick and had never been in the hospital except for kidney stones. Each year my bronchitis kept getting worse, as did my cough. I shrugged it off and just kept taking medicine for the breathing. My breathing worsened to the point that, by the end of the 1990's, I was forced to use a nebulizer and hand-held inhalers daily.

Then the doctor told me the news. I had COPD. I am a college educated person; however, I had no idea what COPD is. In fact, I had never heard of it. I was relieved that it was not cancer. I was relieved I wouldn't have to go through what my mother and all of my aunts and uncles had gone through. My ignorance on the subject would almost result in my demise. For some reason, I did not want to find out any further information on COPD. I wanted to smoke. So I did. The COPD got progressively worse, especially since I had not stopped smoking. Finally, around the year 2004, my breathing had caused me so many problems I was able to quit smoking. Don't get me wrong. I did not want to quit. I did, however, realize that I could not exist any longer in the same mode. They say it's never too late to quit but, for me, it was. One winter night I was going to take my youngest son, Ryan, to the store. When we walked out into the extreme cold and blustery wind, my lungs locked up. I could not get any breaths in or out of my body. I did not freak out but I thought all was over. I lost all of my bodily fluids. My son ran to get my wife to call 911. It's funny what runs through one's mind in a time like this. I did not think about dying. The only thing I thought about was that my wife was going to kick my butt for peeing in my shoes.

The 911 call enabled the First Aid crew to take me to our local hospital for help. There I met two doctors to whom I will always be eternally grateful: Dr. Art Roberson and Dr. John White. They got me through some rough times. I was in this hospital for several weeks and was on 6 liters of oxygen while at rest. I had become about 80 percent bedridden. The only time I would get out of the bed was to go the bathroom. I refused to get help with that. I was scared to get out of the bed and had to wear a PulseOx on my finger at all times so that my oxygen levels could be monitored. I was not in good shape. A drug was used to relax and calm me and keep me from the suffering that goes along with COPD. It sure worked. I told my wife the clock was running backwards. I called one of my step-sons, Austin, "George", and I told my wife the room was full of bugs. I was totally out of it. The hospital was doing everything possible to make me comfortable. I was on a sherbet kick and was given as much sherbet as I wanted. Twice, I had eaten so much there was no more sherbet left in the hospital cafeteria. After I would go on my sherbet binges, I'd simply be given an insulin shot to bring my blood sugar back within normal limits. They knew my time was short and Dr. Roberson had told me so. He is a wonderful man. After he told me I did not have long to live, he hugged me with all of his might. I will never forget that feeling. I truly love that man!! Since that time, we have become good friends. To show what kind of a man he is and to show his sense of humor, I received the following email from him recently: "I have two friends named Harry. They both got a lung transplant. Glad I'm named Art." That's priceless!!

I have been a sports enthusiast all of my life. I played all sports and truly loved golf. At that point in my life, I was still coaching boys' basketball in a recreation league. I just love sports but, at that point, all sports activities had ceased. I became a recluse to the bed or the couch. My productive days were over. I had always been a very independent person. Now, I depended on my family for everything. My step-sons, Austin and Colin Huff, were instrumental in helping me with my oxygen or whatever I needed. My house is a 2-story Colonial and it literally took me 10 minutes to walk upstairs, even with help. I spent many weeks in the hospital and actually went back several times before Dr. White put me in touch with a doctor at Duke Medical Center. After several trips to Durham, NC, and back, my wife called the contact at Duke one day and said, "My husband is dying. You have to help him now." My wife was told to drive me to Duke Medical Center immediately. This is a 3 ½ hour trip from where we lived in Christiansburg, VA. At that point I was on oxygen 24 hours a day which meant she had to get the tanks arranged for the trip. She knew I would freak out about leaving home like this because I had not been off of the couch in several months. I was afraid. The doctor told my wife to give me enough medication to sedate me and to drive me to the Duke Medical Center Emergency Room, and leave me there. This was not mean on anyone's behalf. Their plan was to get me into the hospital quickly to be evaluated. That is, in fact, exactly what happened. She managed to get me there and told them she was leaving me there for evaluation. She then went home. When I awoke the next morning, I had no idea where I was. I was scared. The time of year was almost Christmas, 2009. That morning I was surprised to get a visit from 3 doctors, a social worker, a financial representative, and a coordinator. They explained everything in great detail, I was overwhelmed. I was happy to know where I was and to find out they wanted to help me.

There are many tests to take before undergoing a transplant. A transplant can not be performed on someone who has other critical problems such as cancer. There are lots of obstacles along the way though, for good reason. Some of the procedures one must have are a heart catheterization, a heart scan, a lung scan, pulmonary function tests, numerous blood tests, an echocardiogram, a CT scan, and any other tests deemed necessary. The reason I mention all of these tests is to simply make perfectly clear the fact that the wonderful people involved with saving my life really know what they are doing. They leave nothing for chance. Every last detail is covered. One has to also provide proof of insurance, and dealing with insurance companies on matters like this is tough. They know how much they will have to pay and approval sometimes takes a while. I, plus several of my buddies, had this same problem. Persistence and determination go a long way to fix this problem. Once all of the tests had been completed, I received a return visit from the team that had been there previously. They explained to me that all of my test results were good, except, of course, the lung tests. They also spoke the words I had prayed to hear, "You are eligible for a transplant". They said that I needed to get into the pre-transplant rehab program immediately. I asked one of the doctors how long I had to live, and without missing a beat, he looked at me and said, "6 months at the best". I appreciated his honesty very much. I tried not to, but I cried.

One of the doctors on the team that visited me was Dr. Roy Pleasants. He is very involved with the COPD research in the state of North Carolina, as well as nationally and internationally. We seemed to hit it off pretty well. I respected him very much.

He asked me if I would like to become the face of COPD on billboards in North Carolina. I told him I would do anything I could to help. The offer did, in fact, materialize, and on the billboard was a picture of a pig and me wearing oxygen. The slogan read, "Smoke a pig, not a cig." This relationship with Dr. Pleasants would later lead to my getting involved with making speeches on COPD and transplant awareness.

A major requirement to having a transplant is that one has a full-time caregiver. For obvious reasons, one must move close to the Durham area. After much thought, we decided that my oldest son, Zach, would be my caregiver. My wife had two sons still in school so leaving them to stay with me would not have been practical. I have three other children. My daughter, Kristin, is married with two children. My two youngest sons, Brock and Ryan, couldn't act as caregivers because they were still in school. Zach was my lifeline and did everything for me. I can never repay him for all that he did. Let me say this again. I would not be here today were it not for Zach!! I always say that Ryan saved my life that first night and Zach saved it this time. I'm so very lucky to have such a wonderful family!!! Zach actually quit his job to take care of me. He lived in Winston-Salem at the time. So, when I first started going to rehab, I stayed with him and we drove to Durham every day.

At the time I didn't realize it, but going to rehab changed my life in more ways than I would have imagined. The obvious benefits of rehab were to help us get ready for surgery. There were probably about 20 people in the rehab program when I started. They were all there because they had end-stage lung disease. Some of the different diseases were COPD, Idiopathic Pulmonary Fibrosis, Cystic Fibrosis, Pulmonary Hypertension, and a few others. The rehab program consisted of an exercise regimen and classes. The classes were to educate us on all aspects of the transplant process and were instrumental in our understanding of things to come. They explained that there may be a feeding tube, a tracheotomy, and other subjects such as this. The amount of information to learn was overwhelming.

That's where Zach stepped in and helped me so much. Things I couldn't remember he always did. He was my right arm. The other part of the rehab program was exercising. This consisted of a 5-day a week program for 23 days where we walked for 20 to 30 minutes a day, rode a stationary bike for 20 minutes a day, did some floor exercises and light strength training with weights. Of course, they provided oxygen for us to use while we were there. For any regular person, these exercises were nothing. For someone who can't breathe, they were tough. In the end, I learned these exercises really played a significant part in my recovery.

As I mentioned earlier, rehab changed my life in more ways than one. I cherish the relationships I made there more than anything! I can't explain why but everyone who had a transplant in the same timeframe I did holds a special place in my heart and life. We have developed a bond that will never be broken. I love them all dearly and we keep in touch. When we see each other we cry and hug. My response to all this is simply amazing to me because I've never been an outwardly emotional person, but this experience has changed that. If anything happens to any of these people, it's like it happens to me. We all feel that way. Besides the fellow transplantees, the staff at the Center for Living is awesome. I feel the same way about them as well. I truly love them and appreciate what they do for all of us. Working with people who are complaining that they can not breathe is not easy but they do a remarkable job. They are truly gifted people. I can never repay them either for all they have done for me and my transplant friends!

I finally completed the pre-transplant rehab program and was placed on the transplant list. At the time, I moved to an apartment in Durham so I would be close when they called. Knowing one could receive a call from the Transplant Coordinator at any time was both unnerving and calming. I knew the end was close one way or the other. Every time my cell phone rang, my heart jumped. Probably the toughest parts of this whole ordeal were the dry runs. A "dry run" is when one is on the transplant list and one is called by the Transplant Coordinator to come to the hospital for the transplant. Then for some reason the lungs are determined not to be good enough for transplant and one is sent home. I'm glad the organs are screened so well, but the process worked on me mentally. I had three Dry Runs before I received the fourth call on March 27, 2010, about one o'clock in the morning. I had been on the Transplant List for only 19 days. The coordinator called me and said there was a set of lungs and wanted me to get there right away. We had waited in the hospital for about 12 hours with no word yet on when the surgery would be. I was scared. I told my wife, if this one did not work and was a dry run, then take me home and let me die. I had had enough.

Thankfully, that night about ten o'clock they came to get me to take me to the operating room. As luck would have it, my wife, Sherri, my daughter, Kristin, my sister, Valerie, and all of my sons, Zach, Brock, and Ryan, were there when they took me away. We did a quick group prayer. I was nervous and very apprehensive. I was ready!

I remember the operating room being such a bright place where everything was extremely clean. That made me feel so good. There were about 6 people in the room when I arrived and they were working non-stop. I teased with the anesthesiologist and told her, if everything worked out, I would take them all out for dinner soon. That's the last thing I remember until I woke up in the ICU. The operation had taken about 9 hours, and they repaired a hole in my heart as well. The operation was performed by Dr. Shu Lin, a truly remarkable man. This man saved my life!!! What else can be said about someone like that? One of my heroes in life! This man seeks no credit and is one of the most humble men I have ever met. He's simply a remarkable person! When I did wake, I had an IV in my neck and one in each arm. I had five drainage tubes coming out of my chest, a catheter, and 75 staples holding my chest together. I had wire wrapped around my breastbone holding it together where it had been cut. I had a ventilator tube down my throat yet I was the happiest man in town. I was still alive!! I could not believe how blessed I was.

The first thing I remember, even before I was fully awake, was my nurse telling me not to bite on the ventilator tube. She was right. I chipped off my two bottom front teeth. I also remember thinking, *if you don't want me biting this thing, then take it out.* That day happened to be my youngest son's birthday. The first thing I remember doing in ICU, when I was fully awake, was singing happy birthday to him. We now have the same birthday! I first met Dr. Alan Simeon in the ICU. He came to talk to me about coughing up stuff out of my new lungs and to give me a Bronchoscopy. In the hospital, one is given a Bronchoscopy without any medication or anesthesia. Wow! That's rough, very rough. He told me that, unless I wanted one every day, I had to get up and start walking immediately and start coughing up stuff. He told me in a nice and caring way that made me realize he was thinking about my best interests. I credit him with getting me started on the right foot. I did not want to have to go through that every day. I immediately got up and, with the help of many people, began walking around the ICU halls.

At this point I have to say something about my donor and his or her family. I do not know who they are or anything about them, but I, with all my heart and soul, want to thank them again for giving me a second chance at life. I wrote my donor's family a letter but I have not heard back from them. I would not ever say what was relayed in my letter because it's a personal thing between them and me. Having loved ones myself, I can only imagine how hard going through that process must be. I can only wish the best for them and hope to meet them someday! I am and will always be eternally grateful!

One of the saddest events of my life happened when I was in ICU. One of my buddies from rehab, Ed Brooks, had his transplant about four days ahead of me. I happened to be with him at rehab when he got the call to come to the hospital. I will never forget it. His beautiful wife, Brenda, was so happy, as were the rest of us. Everyone pulled for each other. Ed had a few complications in ICU but seemed to be taking a turn for the better. I saw him the first time I walked and we just looked at each other and smiled. That night I knew something was wrong. My nurse kept coming in and out of my room with a very distressed look on his face. Usually, they stay with you every minute. I also kept seeing Brenda walk past my room. She purposely would not look at me and now I know why. I had a feeling. I told my nurse not to worry about me that I was fine. I told him to please go help Ed. As hard as they tried to save him, Ed took a major turn for the worse and died that night. When I found out, I was devastated. I had just seen him, just smiled at him, just been through rehab with him, and now he was gone. I cried.

I was lucky and was in ICU for only two days. They took me to the step-down floor where I continued to recuperate. After six days, I was released from the hospital. I was scared to leave but they reassured me I was able to leave. After the transplant, one has to go through another 23 days of rehab at the Center for Living. I was released from the hospital on a Friday. Courtney Frankel, a physical therapist at the Center for Living, came in on her off day, Saturday, to get me started back into rehab. I will always be grateful to Courtney for that and for how she and all the other CFL folks treated me. Like I said earlier, these people are my family now!! This round of rehab was better and much easier than the first round. I could breathe now and did not have the anxiety about the operation and the like. What a great concept they have here. They put people who have not had the transplant with the people who have had it so they can see how well we are now doing. Doing so really helps the beginners. Doing so certainly helped me when I started.

After my 23 days of rehab, I went back to Virginia. I hadn't been home in six months and oh, what a thrill to get home. I have been so very lucky in this process and have had so few problems. I have had rejection twice, but it was cleared up both times. I had fluid on my right lung twice, but that was cleared up as well. With the fluid, the first time they took it out they numbed me in the right back area with a local anesthesia and then took a long needle and removed the fluid. I made the mistake of turning around and seeing the needle. Wow was it long! I thought about running but I was being held down. The procedure didn't take that long and really wasn't that bad. The second time I was admitted into the hospital and a drainage tube was placed in my back for several days. I have had no problems with fluid since. The only problem I have now is the Prednisone loves me and I have gained over 25 pounds, all in my neck and stomach. I'll get it off eventually. I am back to work full-time because I feel that will help me live longer and have a better quality of life. I am also back to coaching a boys' basketball team in the recreation league. Our team name is the Young Lungs. I truly feel, if I stayed at home and lay around, I would die much sooner. I have too much to do to die right now. I personally think there are three reasons why I was able to do so well in this endeavor: the doctors, the rehab program, and the transplant coordinators. The doctors with whom I worked are nothing short of outstanding. They all know what they are doing and go about their business in a highly professional manner. They will do whatever they have to at any time. For instance, my operation took nine hours and they began at 10 p.m. on a Saturday night. Following my transplant, they transplanted two of my friends on the same night. Nothing but dedication can get a person through this. As I mentioned earlier, without the rehab at the Center for Living, I don't think the program would be as successful. These people are wonderful. Possibly the most important links in this chain are the transplant coordinators. My post-transplant coordinator is a lady named Cindy Lawrence. She is the ultimate coordinator. She knows her stuff, is on top of everything, and has a great personality. She is my lifeline. If I have any problems or need anything, she is the one I call. Like several others, I can never repay her for all she has done for me!

On one of my return visits to Clinic for a checkup with Dr. Scott Palmer, my transplant pulmonologist and good friend, I noticed a flyer for an organization called the Lung Transplant Foundation (LTF). Dr. Palmer explained that this organization was started by a man named Jeff Goldstein who had a lung transplant several years earlier. This is an organization that raises money for research to try and find a cure for rejection. Fifty percent of lung transplant recipients die within 5 years from chronic rejection. With Dr. Palmer's urging, I contacted Jeff and became involved with the LTF. The people in this organization are wonderful and are simply looking for a way to beat rejection. We want to fix that. We have a vested interest in finding this cure. I give speeches about COPD and transplants in an effort to raise awareness on these subjects. I have been fortunate enough to address the NC Symposium on COPD, the NC Governors Conference on Aging, and the SE Regional Conference on COPD. I truly want to make a difference here and I firmly believe that "Nobody can go back and start a new beginning, but anyone can start today & make a new ending!" That's my new goal in life! I won't be denied!!

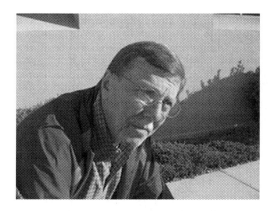

In honor of Robert L. Shanks

How grateful we are to have your story to continue to share it with others throughout the world.

R.I.P.
March 13, 1949 – November 27, 2011

Robert's love for the Lord, perpetual smile, and positive attitude were an encouragement to everyone who knew him. He invested his life well - constantly and lovingly pointing others toward Christ. He loved people and eagerly shared God's grace with anyone who crossed his path.

Many thanks to the amazing doctors and nurses at Duke for giving us this extra year and a half with the miracle of a new lung. To have this time to love and learn from Robert has been a blessing. We will be forever grateful.

Ashley Shanks

# REFLECTIONS FROM MY LUNG TRANSPLANT EXPERIENCE

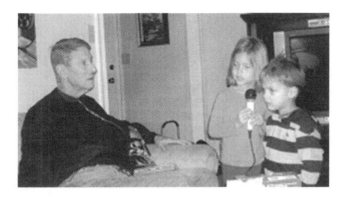

*A Story of God's Grace*

Early in July 2009, Ashley and I caught a virus that affected our respiratory systems. Ashley got over hers in a couple of weeks but mine did not go away, so I went to my doctor. After treatment with antibiotics, I started to get a little better but I had shortness of breath and a cough.

Early in September, our daughter-in-law, Kim Shanks, an allergy and immunology doctor, recommended that I see a pulmonary doctor. The doctor did a CT scan and diagnosed IPF, Idiopathic (cause unknown) Pulmonary Fibrosis. This disease causes lungs to progressively harden, causing a loss of oxygen and $CO_2$ transport from the blood. Not long after, I was admitted to *Duke University Hospital*, one of the best centers for treating pulmonary diseases.

Throughout the Fall, I underwent many tests, which resulted in my being admitted to the Duke Transplant Program on January 4, 2010. I received the miraculous gift of a new lung on February 4, 2010. All during this time I have had the opportunity to reflect on life and the fact that there is a spiritual reality that transcends the physical.

I pray that what I write will be an encouragement to you, and my hope is that you will pass it along to anyone whom you feel may benefit. In addition, please let me know if you or anyone else would like to discuss these things or you think that my story could be a help to someone.

## WHAT IS MY FOUNDATION?

Going into a situation (death of a close friend or family member, emotional crisis, financial crisis/loss of job, etc.) similar to my IPF illness without having as the foundation of your life that you are God's creation, that He created you for a purpose and, regardless of the circumstances, He loves you and is in control, is very difficult. My observation is that, if someone puts off dealing with the reality of God as the foundation of his or her life, then, when a crisis occurs, the person can become afraid, bitter, and doubt can creep in, leading to despair. The person begins asking WHY questions that will not be answered until God is faced (Why do bad things happen to good people?). We do not have to look very far to see that there are a lot of bad things that happen in this world. Natural disasters, sickness/death, innocent people being hurt. Our experience shows us and the Bible is full of examples (Moses, David, and Lot,) of people dealing with all of these and more.

So what is the foundation? The creation story in Genesis describes for us a very special place that God created with variety, beauty, and order (not chaos) and He said it was "good." And, when He created man and woman (mankind), He said they were "very good." They were created in His image, were to enjoy the whole of creation, and were given a free will to make decisions.

106

God did not create robots but rather complex (physically and emotionally) human beings that had purpose, a soul, the ability to choose, and the inherent understanding of what was right and what was wrong. You do not need to read very much further to see that men with free will chose to deceive, envy, kill, and take matters into their own hands. Sin came into the creation. But, God did not give up on creation and mankind because we read that "God is Love" and desires more than anything to have a relationship with each person. However, there is no sin in God, for He and Heaven are perfect. God cannot ignore sin, and when you consider that He loves us and hates sin, you can understand that something radical had to happen. That radical act occurred when Jesus Christ came to earth in the form of man. He lived a perfect life and in one of the mysteries of Heaven, He shed His blood for the remission (forgiveness) of sin. The ultimate price was paid and to prove it He arose from the dead and is in Heaven today looking down and caring for us. Jesus Christ, God's own Son, has been at the center of redemption since the beginning of creation.

I have experienced this renewal of faith and this foundation of faith through the ups and downs of life.

In 1968, my father was killed in Vietnam. In 1986, I lost my job after we had just completed building a new house. In 1992, I had a cancer surgically removed from my tongue. I was diagnosed with IPF in 2009. God has sustained me and my family through all of these circumstances. My foundation has been and is now based on the Biblical account of God's working throughout human history and I accept it by faith. I do not think that my faith is misguided or unreasonable since the Bible describes what I observe in the world today, has stood the test of time, describes the God who created me, loves me, desires a relationship with me, and has provided the way through His Son, Jesus Christ. This free gift of a personal relationship with God is available to all who will believe on Him as their Lord and Savior.

# WHAT IS THE PEACE THE BIBLE DESCRIBES AS "SURPASSING ALL UNDERSTANDING?

I can honestly say that over these past months I have not been apprehensive or nervous about my condition. I have not played "mind games" with myself; rather I have rested in the knowledge that, if God can save my eternal soul, then He can certainly take care of this medical condition. I know that one day I will die and face my Maker. Ashley and I have had honest conversations about the severity of my illness, the lung transplant, organ rejection and the fact that I could die. I was willing to accept that based on God's promises through Jesus's sacrifice for my sins and not my own merit. I tried never to presume that God would take all of this medical condition away and make everything easy. However, His leading us down a clear path was confirmed over and over through so many small and big details. As I experienced Him going before us, that He was in control and I did not have to worry or fret was reaffirmed to me.

An example of this would be that three years ago our son, Brad, moved to Atlanta. Mutual friends encouraged him and a girl he had known at the University of Georgia, Kimsey Smart, to reacquaint. One year later they were engaged and then later that year married, uniting us with Kimsey's mother and father, Bob and Emma Smart and their wonderful extended family. Bob and Emma live in Durham, N.C. On the day that I was diagnosed with IPF, they were visiting a doctor friend in New York. Kimsey called her mother to tell her about me. She in turn told their physician friend. The friend responded that one of his good friends is in the Pulmonary Department at *Duke University Hospital. H*e had that friend's cell phone number and called him immediately. Ten days later I had my first appointment at Duke.

This is just one example of many, many times when God so apparently knew about this illness long before we did and prepared the way for me to be treated. We all have taken great comfort in that and have rested in a peace that passes all understanding.

# PRAYER IS POWERFUL.

I have prayed to God throughout my whole life, but after this experience, I have witnessed and been the recipient of real Prayer Warriors efforts. At first, I was a little uncomfortable with being the center of so much attention. Then I began to understand that so many people were genuinely concerned and were much more consistent and purposeful in their prayer lives. I was convicted of my inconsistent prayer life. To be honest, I think there have been times when I have thought that, if I pray about something a time or two, then God knows about it and will take care of the situation. But, the fact is a lot of people who do not even know me have been praying consistently for me and for specific prayer requests that we have made. Yes, God did know about my illness long before I did, but Jesus, who is God, prayed when He was on earth and He told his disciples to pray. To me, the question is one of those mysteries that will be answered when we are in Heaven. In the meantime, I know that all of these prayers on my behalf have been answered in my human experience. My desire is to be much more purposeful and consistent in my prayer life, knowing that He will teach me more of His purposes and plans and to rest in Him.

# OUR HUMAN BODIES ARE "FEARFULLY AND WONDERFULLY MADE." PSALM 139:13-16

After undergoing all of the preliminary tests to determine if I was eligible for a lung transplant, the doctors determined that all of the other parts of my body were in good shape except for the lungs. I remember being very thankful for this and that thankfulness caused me to thank God for the body that He gave me. Yes, it has flaws and is not the perfect shape, but it has served me very well for all of these years. Although it will deteriorate with time, I have a responsibility to take care of my body, and now in particular, to take care of this gift of a new lung.

Our culture today portrays the perfect physical body. Many times we fall into the trap of comparing ourselves to these unrealistic, and often unhealthy examples, by focusing on our flaws and inadequacies. God knew us before we were even conceived and created us as unique individuals inside and out. To maintain a healthy physical and emotional body, we must be purposeful in caring for both. That means that we must live every moment knowing that God has a purpose for us, and as we pray for his direction, seek out those opportunities that He gives us to serve him and our fellow man. We find true inner joy as we give ourselves away to others. But there must be balance, for if we give ourselves away to the point of ignoring our physical health, then our bodies will suffer. We have a responsibility to take care of our physical bodies. Practically, this means eating correctly (particularly controlling carbohydrates and sugar), maintaining a healthy weight (know what your healthy weight is and focus on that and not body shape), and exercise (this is probably the hardest thing to do, but you must find some exercise that you can do consistently and not make excuses).

Even with my efforts to maintain a healthy body, I got IPF disease. What I have learned about how our bodies work has caused me to be in awe of God's design. And, being the recipient of the skillful and wonderful care that I have received at *Duke University Hospital* has caused me to be in awe of God's gifts to doctors and nurses. When people with skill, knowledge, and compassion realize that they have been given these gifts from God, they are a true blessing physically and emotionally to those that they treat because they give hope for today and for eternity. I have met many doctors and nurses at Duke that, when I say, "I have received a true miracle from God," they respond, "Yes, you have."

And finally, there is the issue of the donor. I have to admit that early on I was so self-centered that I never gave serious thought to the donor family and the person who would make possible my lung transplant. Before my transplant, I received an e-mail from our good friends Dottie and Mike Fitzhenry and they said that we should be praying for this family. I shared this on my *Caringbridge* site and Linda Tucciarone of *Heritage Academy* put it in perspective by writing that the donor and family are making "A living sacrifice to give life through their death." She drew the parallel to how Christ gave us eternal life by His death on the

Cross. I have not been the same since and pray every day for this family. Protocol requires that one year pass before the donor and recipient can contact each other. We have heard wonderful stories of these contacts and I pray that will be the case with us because I could not have survived if I had not received this lung. What a wonderful and miraculous gift. I would encourage everyone to be an organ donor if you are not already.

I do have one last thought. Ashley's and my relationship has always been supportive and loving. This experience has only brought us closer together. She is not only my wife, but my soul mate, and now my "primary caregiver." She and I together have been blessed with four (our two sons and their wives) wonderful children, so many special friends, and family that have been such an encouragement through their prayers, gifts, and time with us. We are eternally grateful.

Thank you for taking the time to read my thoughts. I hope that they are an encouragement to you and to anyone who reads them. Praise be to God!!

Ashley Shanks        E-mail: ashrobshanks@hotmail.com
33 Indian Cove Rd      Phone: Home 706-736-4894
Augusta, Ga. 30909

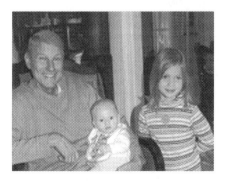

# Living Fully With Cystic Fibrosis

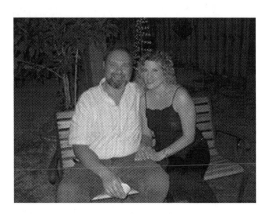

## *A Story of Self Discovery and Acceptance*

At age 48 I mostly feel victorious living with Cystic Fibrosis (CF), even though today marks six weeks since my double lung transplant. It's all part of my journey. My message is living a full, joyful life is possible with CF.

Diagnosed at two months old by a sweat test, the doctors knew to suspect CF since I had two siblings with it. Four years later, my younger brother, Mark, was also diagnosed with CF. His diagnosis made four out of four kids, unlikely odds given that there was only a 25% chance each child would have CF.

I lost my older brother, Ricky, when he was 14 years old and my sister, Cindy, when she was four months.

I remember vividly the moment I chose to take charge of my disease: My parents were telling Mark and me that Ricky had died. I did the math in my head and said to myself, "Ricky is 14, and I'm ten. I have four years to live. Hell no! This disease isn't going to get me!"

Lucky for us, our parents were willing to do everything medically recommended and more for our well-being. Thus, when I was five they left everything they ever knew and we moved from Michigan to Florida because warm coastal air was highly recommended. They learned chest physiotherapy (CPT), mist tent, medications, diet, supplements, exercises, et cetera. We worked as a team, on a firm schedule, to fit everything an average family does, plus our medical regimens.

Before school, I'd rise from my soggy bed, wet from sleeping in my mist tent, to keep my lung secretions moist and loose, easier to expectorate. Then I'd take my nebulized bronchodilator, readying myself for my parents to do chest physiotherapy for 30 minutes. This treatment shook the mucus loose and made raising secretions easier. I didn't like having to do CPT as a kid yet I'm ever grateful to my parents for doing it to keep my lungs clear and make CPT a non-negotiable necessity. As an adult, when I became highly productive with sputum, CPT was much easier to accept as part of my routine.

Mom made special high-calorie, low-fat, home-made food. Sometimes we were on strict diets making cooking especially challenging for her. I remember for my 17th birthday, when I couldn't eat wheat, she made a rice flour cake. It looked beautiful and it tasted like a garbage can; we had so many laughs over that.

I was a tom-boyish kid, naturally active and enrolled in various classes and sports: cheerleading, gymnastics, volleyball, dancing, swimming and diving. Exercising was key in keeping my lungs healthy and cleared. Running was an adjunct to CPT.

In fact, when I went an hour away to college and stayed in the dorm, I did one CPT with a hand-held percussor and, instead of a second therapy, I'd run a mile or two. That hand-held percussor was actually a converted (with a pad) Black & Decker jigsaw. That percussor really got the mucus moving. After freshman year, I got rid of the mist tent since my doctor believed then that keeping the mist tent clean was a liability outweighing its' benefit. I felt triumphant going to college, managing independently of my parents and feeling well. Luckily, in my second semester I decided on a major—nursing. Well, summer school was necessary to keep pace with my class. So, a friend and I stayed off campus with an older lady who allowed us to do house work to pay for our room. Not having a car, I had to ride my bike nine miles to class, which was exhilarating.

Scuba diving was one of the most fun and contributing elective courses I took. Too bad it was in January . . . brrrr. Each success or new endeavor lifted me and I gained confidence.

However, for the first time since childhood, I experienced hospitalization during my sophomore year. I was to rest, take extra chest physiotherapy sessions and have various tests; my doctor didn't order any IV antibiotic therapy that stay. About ten days later I was back on top. The next two years I coasted, having fun, doing what I needed for my health and focusing on nursing until graduation.

Soon after graduation, I got a job at Jackson Memorial Hospital (J.M.H.) in Miami on the general medical floor's 3-11 shift. My goal was to learn as much as I could as fast as I could and, given it is a major teaching hospital, J.M.H. delivered. About a year and a half into nursing, I found the job real tiring. I noticed I was short of breath just changing a patient's bed. I thought, *I need a change*. One change was hiring a respiratory therapist to do my CPT a few times a week. Also, after consulting my head nurse, she encouraged me to interview for a position that had just become available in Community Health Education. Two interviews later I had the job. First, I learned the ropes. Then, I managed, designed, and implemented the programs aboard the Health Care-a-Van, a 32-foot Winnebago used by the hospital to educate the public and provide health screening at various locales in the community.

After six years, my body was protesting. I had recurring fevers, fatigue, and congestion, even after steadily increasing my CPT session with the therapist to twice a day. My usual biannual "tune-ups" (aka two week hospital stays for CF exacerbation) turned into three or four times per year. Again, something had to change. My administrator let me first try part-time work, then, telecommuting, until I had to make one of the toughest decisions of my life—to retire.

I became a nurse with one patient, my self. My job was my health. My health routine took six hours a day: three hourly CPT sessions, nebulizers, exercise, and naps. In 1990, two years before retiring, I was married. Having a partner in life made this transition so much easier. I did struggle, though. I was so used to believing that my worth was equal to my productivity. What was I doing and how could I tally my worth?

Enter my spiritual path. I expanded my mind and was on a journey to find peace, a slower pace, and learn to exalt in my slower pace.

I traveled a lot, promising myself to go to a different county or destination per year. My favorite trip was a ten day dive trip in the Galapagos Islands. Good planning was required for travel. I'd take a respiratory therapist, rent oxygen, and take my therapy equipment and loads of medication.

I volunteered for the CF Foundation and Cystic Fibrosis Foundation of Florida. I helped form the Cystic Fibrosis Alliance, Inc., a non-profit organization committed to having medical insurance security for all CF patients. Our greatest feat was getting Florida to create a supplementary insurance for uninsured or underinsured CF patients. I also continued my work with the United States Adult Cystic Fibrosis Association (U.S.A.C.F.A.) which produced a quarterly newsletter called The CF Roundtable

(CFR). The CFR was a newsletter written by CF adults for CF adults nationwide.

The next couple of decades wore slowly on me with some bumps in the road. I was divorced. I experienced my first life-threatening complication of CF, called massive hemoptysis (coughing up blood). Consequently, I was hospitalized; my conditions were touch and go, including a couple bronchial arterial embolization procedures to stop the bleeding. After a month, I was discharged with continuous-running oxygen. I always believed in my strength and ability to overcome, however, I had a difficult time not feeling defeated. I felt weak, unpredictable, and at the effect of my disease for the first time. I felt the disease had me instead of me having the disease.

What? Me? I'm the one who has controlled my disease up to now. My CPT sessions were altered from my usual "aggressive" style to "light" without Trendelenberg (aka postural drainage in a 45 degree angle downward) positions, all to discourage another bleed. Months later, finally the danger of a recurrent bleed ceased and I returned to aggressive CPT. After doing "light" CPT for those months, I became filled with secretions and really had a lot of work to return to good health.

I was prescribed an eight week pulmonary rehabilitation program to regain my pulmonary status and strength. Not only did the program work wonders, I felt well enough to start a pulmonary support group with the help of another nurse.

I no longer needed continuous oxygen, only during sleep and exercise. As a safety net, I enrolled in a lung transplant program in Miami. Happily, I was deemed "too healthy". As a result of creating a pulmonary support group for the hospital, I was featured in a weekly community newspaper. From that article, along with my desire to write, I approached the publisher to ask if I could work for her. She hired me on the spot, saying that she like that I had no experience in journalism and she would edit my work. I popped out of her office on top of the world and ready to delve into reporting and writing by immersion. I wrote for 18 months until my disease required more of my attention.

The next couple years I was on and off oxygen and mostly homebound. I would fatigue more. And I was diagnosed with pulmonary hypertension. Slowly, after being told by my trusted doctor in 2005 that I was ready for a lung transplant and I probably would not get off the oxygen, I realized that I really needed to look into a lung transplant. I did inform the transplant doctors that I'm the "come back kid" and plan to get off the oxygen and not be a candidate. I was true to my word, putting off my transplant . . . until 2011.

In 2006, I met the love of my life, Steve. Life's sweet pleasure!

Here I write, at age 48, a month and a half after my successful transplant at Duke University Hospital. Breathing freely, feeling energized wanting to give hope and health to all that need to hear. I've been granted another chance, a *rebirthday*!

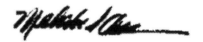

# EN ROUTE TO A TRANSPLANT . . . DESTINATION REACHED 11/11/11

# Pulmonary Journey

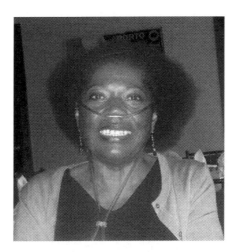

## *A Story of hope*

"Mrs. Price, we have done some preliminary tests and you have something going on in your lungs, but we don't know what; more tests are needed. Did you say your insurance carrier was Kaiser Permanente? Okay, we're going to send you over to University of North Carolina Hospital (UNC). They are the Kaiser HMO hospital."

Making that statement, Dr A. studied the chart, more closely than necessary it seemed to me, for she already knew what was there. The news was bad. She wouldn't make eye contact. Dr A. was a senior resident with whom I had bonded over the course of a few hours in the Duke University Medical Center Emergency Department. Through the frightful twisting, turning, poking, prodding, and bloodletting that are standard procedure for one entering the ED with an apparent life-threatening situation, with care and concern she had explained each step of testing and diagnosis. That we had discovered we had a mutual friend was of no comfort to me as my heart slammed in my chest and the bottom dropped from my stomach. The feeling that had subsided a bit since arriving at the ED was now back with a vengeance. Dr. A's words floated toward me diffused and milky, like an early morning sun pushing through a pea-soup fog. I was scared. Petrified. "What? You don't know what's wrong with me?"

I fought the stupor that had enveloped my entire awareness, to find purchase. The words formed in my brain but did not translate into the questions I was struggling to ask. Surely there was a drug, a cocktail of medications, to treat conditions like mine. Right? Mentally, I packed up to go back home. The gauzy green curtains meant to provide a modicum of privacy began to advance toward me, suffocating me in their antiseptically nauseating cocoon. I strained to sit up to look at Dr A's face. Another physician, the attending I later learned, materialized beside the bed looking down at me with intense, worried eyes. "Don't move, Mrs. Price. I'll move the back of the bed up. There. That better?" Dr. A. added, "You do not want to put any pressure on your heart. There are pressures building in your lungs and we don't know why. When you get over to UNC Hospital the doctors there will continue to evaluate to find out why the pressures are building". *What were they really telling me? I'm not going to live?*

Always ready to confront life head on, my "can do, I can handle anything" spirit over the last three months had been smashed and replaced with a paralyzing numbness and nothingness. How much more was there for a soul to absorb? In one lucid moment, I had a flash of a thirteen year old boy asleep in his bed. Was BA still sleeping? Maybe. The hour was not yet daybreak. I needed my son to know where I was and to be assured that I was okay. My cousin, Mike, had come over when I called in the middle of the night, and his wife Windy had come along to drive me to the hospital. Kristen, my daughter, had stayed on the coast with my mom. BA and Kristen's well-being were priority one. They'd both been through enough!

We had, just two days before, returned from a five day Caribbean cruise. Our family cruise, the one we planned a year in advance with my parents, sister, cousins and their families, was the most miserable trip of my life. My husband, the love of my life and the father of my children, had passed away a mere two months before. He had so looked forward to the cruise. Backing out wasn't an option for me and the kids, though Lord knows I tried. Grieving stalwartly, I soldiered on, believing primordially my children needed constant activity so as not to dwell on their father's absence from our lives. There was also the fact that losing $2000 with no benefit was not an option. I was thankful that there were a number of children of all ages in our group. I didn't have to babysit my "tweens", the cruise ship was family friendly and kids had special age-specific activities. Oh, we did a little snorkeling and I sat on the deck baking in the 110 degree Caribbean sun while they parasailed across the sky above azure blue water. I participated in all the touristy adventures abounding on the ports of call. No one was aware of how heavy a lift it was for me to show up each day. Besides what my family understood as my grief, I was battling inordinate fatigue, shortness of breath, and an accelerated heartbeat that was leaving me listless, lethargic, and so very afraid. My darkened skin I thought a gift from the fierce Caribbean sun. Not so. It was from oxygen deprivation. Cyanosis, it is called medically. I was turning blue!

Getting back to port in Florida, we drove seven hours to the North Carolina coast in time for the Fourth of July holiday. The next day my son and I drove back home to Durham. The niggling thought that something might be seriously wrong kept bubbling up in my consciousness like the contents of an overheated cauldron. I knew I had to see a doctor soon. I had not slept for two nights, afraid to fall asleep for fear of dying. I snatched naps sitting in bed propped up on a mound of pillows. I hadn't even acknowledged the blackouts that had been occurring with more regularity over the last month. How many times did I come-to, lying on the floor of my bedroom or standing and momentarily fading out and back in? Everything in my being screamed, "Get some help!" Little did I know that I was a ticking time bomb with a life threatening lung disease which was creating pressures that could explode my heart.

I decided late in the night to go to the emergency room. I was sick and afraid. My heart pounded and I couldn't take a complete breath. I was more afraid of what would happen to my children if something happened to me.

The fogginess lifted a bit around the edges of my conscious-ness. The voices of the doctors and assistants prevailed. What had been gibberish in my brain became distinguishable snatches of conversation directed at me. "UNC has an excellent cardiotho-racic program . . ." " . . . we are sending the X-rays and . . . ." "Get pulmonary pressures down . . ." "Some heart failure likely . . .". "Is transport here . . . ?" "Alert the Kaiser doctor that Mrs. Price is on the way . . ."

My numbness was complete. Laying mute, a battalion of nurses and assistants thronged around me in efficient practiced movements preparing me for travel. The preparation was as intense as prepping for surgery. Finally, I was unhooked and unconnected, then moved onto a gurney and rehooked and reconnected to life sustaining oxygen and IV solutions for my trip to UNC Hospital.

## At University of North Carolina Hospital

Dr. Namita Sood was a highly regarded pulmonary fellow and had been on my case exclusively, it seemed, since I had been admitted.

"Pulmonary Hypertension" was the diagnosis.

A heart catheterization had given Dr. Sood the verification that she had diagnosed correctly. Pulmonary Hypertension . . . .

Pressures building in my lungs because of the scarring and stiffness of a disease called Sarcoidosis, where the pulmonary artery would not allow oxygen and blood to flow through easily. They said it was partially occluded. The high pressures caused my heart to pump harder to get blood and oxygen through creating congestive heart failure.

There have been two times in my life when I've had the experience of being totally wrenched from my mooring, a cataclysm that caused intense pain and left me feeling on the edge of nothingness and losing everything that was near and dear to me. The pain was intense and unrelenting. It was emotional, spiritual, and physical. The physical pain was made more acute by my emotional haze.

The weeks following my midnight sojourn to Duke University Medical Center (DUMC) Emergency Department, then to the University of North Carolina (UNC) Hospital on July 5, 1998, unleashed a torrent of silent lethal emotions, a tidal wave of turmoil churning and twisting me down to my miserable core. I engaged as best I could with the doctors, nurses and technicians as I was wheeled from x-ray to MRI to Pulmonary Function to VQ scan, from cardiac catheterization to lip biopsy, trying to hear and absorb the status of my condition by what they were not finding. More telling was the attentiveness to my care as if I were a commodity marked "fragile", requiring only the most sensitive handling lest I shatter. No getting up without help; actually no getting up at all. Day in and day out, a contingent of cardiopulmonary attending physicians, fellows, residents and interns congregated in the room around my bed, filling notebooks of what was heretofore the minutiae of my life, medical and personal. "Did you ever work around chemicals? Have you ever been exposed to asbestos? What kind of work did you do? What is state of your father's health? What is the state of your mother's health? What did your sister die from?" Repetitive questions. Was it that, asked the questions enough times, a picture would emerge that would provide the answers to why and what had run amok in my lungs? Then everyone with a stethoscope listened front, back, up, down, stomach and ankles. Were there pulses in the ankles?

Many days I'd awake to see Dr. Sood leaning against the wall in my room, staring into the far distance as if fathoming the complexities of the universe. That sight in itself was a bit scary to me, a further indication of the severity of my condition.

The tests, the evaluations, the constant attention combined with my internal malaise, made me feel as if my very existence was being threatened. I am by nature an optimist, attacking life's issues by wrestling them to the ground. Whatever I touched came under my submission. This agonizing search for ground, for some stability, was not responsive to my normal *modus operandi* using intellect, reasoning, God, faith, and family. The effort was a desperate one to find a way out and my internal dialogue resembled a hallucinogenic overload of wayward thoughts, never coalescing into coherence and lucidity. A lot of energy spent to no good end.

My story was chronicled in the endless reams of paper that comprised my medical record. That I had just recently lost my husband and now was dealing with a debilitating lung disease with two young children red-flagged my records for the psychiatrist, the psychologist, and the chaplain. The chaplain paid a visit. He was a young African American guy and a recent graduate of where else? UNC-Chapel Hill. He became somewhat of a life line. He made me laugh, something I hadn't done in a while. We had common ground. His wife was in the same sorority as my sister who went to UNC and, since the timing was right, we decided that they probably knew each other. We found also that his mother was from my hometown on the coast of North Carolina and I knew a couple of his aunts. He asked me about the circumstances surrounding my husband's death. I told how details in the aftermath were hazy. I remember a ghostlike existence. I was floating, functioning, performing, participating and making decisions, but never quite feeling. I confided that

I still had not grieved but had only walked further into the fog made more opaque by my illness.

The chaplain made me laugh. He asked me if I had cried, screamed or hollered in my grief. My response was "No. I don't grieve that way". "Oh", he said, "you did the Jackie Kennedy", referring to Jacqueline Kennedy's unblinking, stiff upper lip stoicism during the very public death and burial of her husband, President John F. Kennedy. I laughed. We both knew that funerals in the African American community could be quite entertaining: Hats slinging, hems flying, fallings out and lying on the casket. We both knew people who attended funerals of people they didn't even know, kind of like a pastime or hobby, to see how the family "cut up". The laughter felt good. The pain diminished somewhat.

My days began to take on purpose and I began paying attention. I began to listen and ask questions. Action seemed essential. Even though the deep fear and uncertainty was still there and the options unclear, there was going to be a tomorrow and I had to figure how I was going to fit in it. I was in the hospital at UNC for 21 days. I had lots of time to contemplate my situation. I still struggled frantically, but I knew that, to heal emotionally and physically, I had to look my reality in the face and not shrink from it but know and acknowledge it. I was not there yet. I was searching, looking for ground on which to stand. The physical healing was an experiment with various and sundry therapies, drug regimens and diet. The most recent and advanced therapy for treating PH (Pulmonary Hypertension) was an intravenous drug called Flolan®. Flolan® had shown great promise in trials, and now in PH patients like me. I had surgery to install a Hickman catheter to administer this drug through a cassette attached to a battery-operated pump. With this drug, I was committing to a daily regime of storing, mixing and maintenance, plus all that goes with catheter site maintenance.

I hadn't completely accepted the dire diagnosis and what was to be my way of life. I only knew that I was beginning a long, physical, and emotional journey on an unknown and unfamiliar path. I didn't know where I would end up yet I believed in the power of God and the power of prayer, and wherever that would be, I would be okay.

## Fast forward. April, 2005. Duke University Medical Center

2004 was an active year for me. I worked full-time for Measurement Inc. until July, at which time I began managing the campaign office and volunteers for my sister Wanda Bryant's run for re-election to the North Carolina Court of Appeals. Immediately after the election, my daughter was selected to participate in Alpha Kappa Alpha Sorority's Debutante Cotillion Scholarship Program. I worked relentlessly raising funds, attending meetings, and meeting all of the parental obligations associated with preparing for my daughter's "coming out" debut. On April 5, 2005, the day after the Cotillion Ball, I checked myself into the Duke University Medical Center Emergency Department, subsequently being admitted to the hospital.

Dr T., my pulmonologist, told me that I was one bag of oxygen away from an intubation. Further, he said, if I were intubated, I would most likely never come off of it as that was the nature of my disease. I couldn't get a lung transplant because I was much too overweight. I was, by the charts, obese. Dr T. asked me if my family actually knew how sick I was. I had taken a lot of pains to keep them in the dark, or at least fuzzy about the extent of my condition. I was raising two teen-age, almost-adult children. My son was in his second year of college and my daughter would be graduating from high school in a month with plans for college in the fall. Dr T. spoke with my sister, Wanda, about the slender thread of my existence. How dire the prognosis was.

The stark reality of my medical condition was the beginning of a change in my life and lifestyle that propelled me to November, 2009, when I was referred to the lung transplant office by Dr Terry Fortin. Dr. Fortin told me right after recuperating from the 2005 event that, if I lost weight, she would do the referral for a lung transplant. Between 2006 and 2009, I lost close to 50 pounds. Since that time, I have lost an additional 40 pounds. I began testing and evaluation for lung transplantation in November, 2009, continuing through 2010. September 2011 I met the weight goal, completed all outstanding tests and procedures, signed consent forms and now waiting to get listed for transplant surgery.

My days are focused on strengthening my faith through study and prayer, strengthening my body through healthy eating and exercise, and paying for my transplant surgery through fundraising and investments,

I am what we are calling "en route" to transplant. There is a culture at Duke Center for Living Pulmonary Rehabilitation that makes the striving easier. Many of us are working toward the same goals of either getting ready for a transplant, recuperating after a transplant, working to maintain the new lungs, or learning to live with a chronic lung disease. The hardship and, sometimes hopelessness, fades when a person fellowships, at times commiserates, but mostly becomes motivated by those who are going through just the same. Amazing are those who are pushing a walker with an oxygen tank, struggling for breath yet, when one says, "hello, how are you?", they respond, "I'm great"! No other place would one find that kind of enthusiasm and positiveness. My work toward transplant is made easier. The therapists and staff at the Pulmonary Rehabilitation Program at Duke Center for Living are phenomenal. For them, their work is not merely a job, but an avocation. Each therapist has passion for what he or she does and it is evidenced in their patience and the one-on-one time with each and every patient. They patiently answer our sometimes inane questions, calm our frustrations, encourage us and, yes, push us harder to get the results that they know will be beneficial in the long run.

# SOME BATTLES ARE WON ON THE OTHER SIDE

# Ed Brooks—A Love Song

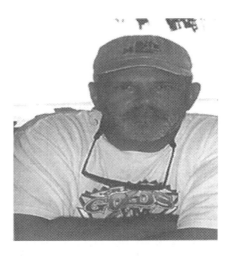

## *A Story of Passion for Life and for Love*

Sitting on our patio in the evenings was always a special place and time for us. There was something magical about it and still is. For years, I had been joking with Ed about writing me a love song. Not only did he have a special way with words, he also played guitar and sang. I thought it appropriate he write a song for me. This particular evening on the patio in July 2009, as we were holding both hands and looking straight into each other's tear filled eyes, he told me not all love songs are written. Some are lived. We had lived the perfect love song, but the last verse was being written now.

Ed was diagnosed with IPF just two months earlier in May 2009. His breathing capabilities had worsened. We were fortunate enough to be able to see Dr. Lake Morrison at Duke as his pulmonologist. Dr. Morrison and the staff were wonderful. We were facing death square in the face with this disease, but they let us know there was hope.

The caregiver role in the transplant process is special. I had been my mother's caregiver before she died, but that had not prepared me for this journey.

Ed was a very active person who loved and lived life to its fullest on a daily basis. To see that person become so limited was very difficult. I was responsible for the mortgage division for a bank that was shut down by the NC Commissioner of Banks (as directed by the FDIC), just a couple months after his diagnosis. As an executive, I lost my job immediately when the new bank that the FDIC chose, took over. Surprisingly, this turned out to be a good thing. Ed had gone downhill so quickly in those couple months I did nothing about seeking other employment and devoted my time to managing his health care. This was the most important job I would ever have. To keep healthy mentally, Ed chose to go to work each day. As the weeks went along, this became more of an ordeal for both of us.

My life became getting him up and helping him get ready for the office. Oxygen had to be loaded in his truck each day sufficient to last him until he could get home. He worked with some amazing people who loved him dearly, and they began waiting for him to pull up in the parking lot and would meet him to carry in the oxygen to his office. During the day I would be getting oxygen deliveries, coordinating doctor appointments as well as taking over all household duties. There were household chores and lawn care that we had always paid others to do but with our income diminished dramatically, I took over those responsibilities. During this time I learned about oxygen and how that could be dispensed. We experimented with many different forms until we hit on something that worked best until his needs increased, and we had to change all over again.

Finally, Ed's lung capacity reached a level that Dr. Morrison thought it time for us to be evaluated for the transplant. It was

November, and we were in Durham for a week of evaluation. I recall how stressful this was and how exhausting. Ed had to pass all the tests to make it through to the next level of treatment, or he would be going home to die. And yet, this was a partnership. I had as much at stake as he did because I thought surely my life would be over if he died. My journal entry for November 13 says in part "I just pray for the strength to be able to be there for him no matter what his needs. The bottom line is I am so scared". In spite of my faith, that scared feeling lurked in the recesses of my mind for some time.

During evaluation week we met some wonderful and amazing people who are still important to me. The closest relationships were formed with other transplant hopefuls, but relationships were also formed with some of the transplant team members. We were back home on Friday to begin the wait for the call of whether we were accepted or not. Tuesday evening before Thanksgiving the phone rang, and I saw it was a 919 area code. My heart was pounding the second I saw the Duke number. We made it! There were stipulations and more hoops to jump through with tests, but we were at least being given a chance. One of the stipulations was that Ed had to lose weight. What a challenge this was since he was on heavy doses of prednisone and couldn't exercise effectively. He was in pulmonary rehab locally but that wasn't helping with weight loss He put all his effort into it though, and we walked inside the house just to move and perhaps burn some calories.

Our diet was modified even more, and Dr. Morrison cut back the milligrams of prednisone to help with the weight loss. By Christmas, he was pretty sick, and I wasn't certain he was going to live long enough to get a transplant. Always, always, always his attitude was positive, and he had a smile on his face. Finally in January 2010, after sufficient weight loss and getting through a couple more medical follow up tests, we were able to move to Durham and begin pre-transplant rehab at the Center for Living. We saw our old friends from evaluation week and forged even stronger bonds with them. When one is going through a life and death journey together those bonds become so strong. I saw a couple people come and go from rehab each day, and sometimes they seemed to want to isolate themselves. I have a hard time understanding that because the comfort in the sharing process was so very important to Ed and me. The blessings we received from getting to know some of those people are still unexplainable. Sometimes it was just a knowing look, a smile or hug. We encouraged each other, worried about each other and rejoiced when someone got "the call" to get their new lungs or any other success.

On February 26, while at the Center for Living, my phone rang, and we got the notice that Ed had been activated. We didn't have to wait long to get the first call to come to the hospital. Of course, we were prepared by the team for dry runs and that first call on March 1st was just that. We were at the hospital about six hours before we were given the word to go back home. The next call took longer and even though it was only 6 days we had our appetite wetted and were ready for a transplant. March 7 at midnight we got another call and by the time we arrived at the hospital we were called to go back home so we didn't even get admitted that time. We got a little sleep and at 9a.m., we were called again. At 6p.m., we were sent back home again. What an emotional roller coaster! We made the decision not to tell family or friends about all these calls until we knew it was a go for surgery, so we were going through all these dry runs alone—except for our transplant family. They shared the joy and disappointment with us because many of them had gone through the same experience.

March 9, 1:45 pm, we received one more call. We left rehab and got home to get our pre-packed bag again and head to the hospital one more time. We went through all the prep again and waited. We waited, and we waited. Remembering things in hind sight that Ed said to me, he knew this was it. At 7:30 pm we were told the lungs were ours, and it was a go. Oh my God! I wanted that call, but now I was scared to death. I was excited. I was happy. I didn't know what to think. Calls now had to be made to family, so they could come to the hospital. In between all the prep, Ed and I shared some soul touching moments until he was whisked off to surgery a little before 10pm. As could be imagined it was a long night, and at 5:30 am Dr. Davis came out to tell me all was well.

All during Ed's illness I had a note taped to my computer screen that said "Do not be afraid of tomorrow for God is already there". Seeing this on a daily basis brought me great comfort especially, during this hospitalization. All was well the first day and night. I was so excited to talk with him, to look into his eyes again and see his love for me, but joy, elation and thankfulness turned into chaos very quickly. He developed a massive thoracic hemorrhage and was sent flying down the hall past me, with doctors and nurses for emergency surgery. I will forever be indebted to his nurse, Jason Gough, for being astute enough to realize in a split second there was a problem and for being my emotional rock at that time. Then, Ed was out of surgery and all was well again. I considered this a setback, but not one we could not overcome. Ed's entire life was spent being athletic and extremely competitive. I knew he would work harder than anyone to get back to normal, or as normal as he could be. The first couple days were great. Walking with him down the hall so soon after two major surgeries was like a miracle to me. All the hope we had was being fulfilled.

After those first couple days, there were so many ups and downs. Anxiety set in for him. He would beg me to stay because he said he could not breathe if I was not there with him. In his delusion, he thought the night nurse was trying to kill him and an assortment of other anxiety issues. He began to develop all sorts of physical problems at this point also. Through it however, he pushed himself to walk because he knew from our classes this was critical to getting well and out of the hospital. That competitive spirit of his was still there, and with some encouragement from me I really thought we could overcome whatever this was. Individually, maybe not, but together there wasn't much we couldn't do. We always had a joke about this in fact. A daily ritual was to do a crossword puzzle together and at its completion one of us would say "together we are something and can do anything".

Ed and I met dancing and were actually quite good during the heyday of two stepping and swing in the early 90's. We even danced competitively and had talked about getting back to dancing as a form of exercise when he had his new lungs. To encourage him to walk, I would assume my dance position in front of him and "two step" backwards down the hall as motivation for him. I won't ever forget that "last dance" we had down the halls of 3200 Duke Hospital. As the song says, "I could have missed the pain but I would have had to miss the dance".

So much happened in the next days and his status deteriorated. The doctors were frustrated because they couldn't "fix" him. If Jason Gough, our nurse, was my rock that second day in the hospital, Dr. Alan Simeone was every day after that. I truly don't know what I would have done without the confidence I felt in him. In addition to the confidence I felt in his knowledge and skill, his compassion for what I was going through and what Ed was going through was immeasurable. I will never, ever forget him. The staff on 3200 and the transplant team were special individuals who deserve all the accolades I can give them.

On March 30 Ed was put on life support to buy time that day to determine if anything could be done to save his life. I sincerely believe everything possible was in fact done to save him but on March 31, but with no more hope, in the early morning hours, I made the decision to discontinue life support. By this time all of Ed's family had gathered at the hospital. My favorite two RN's, Jason Gough and Nicole Martin happened to be working and were there. Dr. Simeone, who I don't think left mine and Ed's side for a couple days, was there also. I nodded at Nicole for her to shut down life support. With the equipment off, silence filled the room. His brother Steve sang one of his favorite songs, Mr. Bojangles, as his life on this earth ended at 8:43am. They allowed us to make his passing a beautiful thing.

I have been asked many times if it was all worth it. The answer is a resounding yes. Remember, I would have had to miss the dance. I do believe Ed would have died by the end of March anyway without the transplant. Because of the journey God sent us on I have met some wonderful people and many of them I now count as my friends. Staying in touch with other transplant patients and families makes my heart sing because of their successes. I find joy in that.

Our transplant story doesn't end with Ed's death. We discussed early on in the rehab phase of our journey about giving back to other transplant patients and families. I have not found my role yet, but I will.

We had a love like none other, together on earth, for 20 years. When he was initially diagnosed, we both knew, just knew, without voicing it, he would not live long, no matter what. I don't believe the last verse of our love song was written though. He made me a better person, and I will use that to continue sharing his love for life and be an example to others to live their lives, really live their lives, every day. The love song will continue.

*Brenda McDonald*
*for my love, Ed Brooks*

# Contributions

## Catherine Lee/Brockington

Catherine Lee/Brockington is the daughter of Charlotte Patterson and the late Arthur V. Patterson. She has four kids two of each and four grandchildren three boys and one darling girl. She spends her time at the Center for living on good days and reading and researching about her lung disease on other days.

## Jim Clary

James B. Clary was born in Gaffney, SC on November 17, 1942. He received a BS and MS in Electrical Engineering from Clemson University and completed his PhD coursework in Electrical Engineering at Duke University. Formally with Bell Telephone Laboratories for 7 years, he retired from the Research Triangle Institute after 23 years, the last 10 of which he served as Research Vice President of the Electronics and Systems business unit. His hobbies include Amateur Radio and gardening.

## Beverly A. Cordes

Beverly Cordes is the daughter of Beatrice Garrett and the late John Garrett Jr. She is the youngest of her 7 siblings. She is the mother of one son Tyler and the grandmother of a seven year old granddaughter. She resides in North Carolina, where she attends pulmonary rehab, spends time advocating for lung disease and living her life to her fullest potential.

## Joan Fox

Joan Fox moved to Durham, NC with her husband Pat in 1994 from Chatham, NJ. She taught Developmental English at Butner prison for 12 years to fill out her retirement years. She is recovering from lung cancer surgery diagnosed in 2010 and enjoys her time at Duke Chapel, the Duke Center for Living and the Treyburn golf course.

## Shirley White

Shirley White migrated from Atlantic City, NJ to Durham, NC to live with her daughter in 2002. Seventy-six years young, she is the mother of six with three boys and three girls. Moving to North Carolina has truly added years to her life, and she continues to travel and live life to the fullest.

## Virginia M. Barnette

Virginia Barnette is a retired registered nurse. She is mother, grandmother, sister and friend. She was diagnosed with the rare disease of sarcoidosis in 1984. She has never lost her smile even though this disease has been elusive and difficult to treat. She is on a mission to educate African Americans who are disproportionately affected by this disease.

## Cassandra (Sam) Adkins

Cassandra (Sam) Adkins is the daughter of Shirley White. She is one out of six children, and is the baby girl in the family. She resides in Durham, NC where her mother lives with her and her husband, and toy poodle Romeo. As the care provider, she manages work, family, and caring for her mother with the help of the good Lord.

## Lorraine Williamson

Lorraine Williamson has resided in North Carolina, for the past ten years, with her husband, Don. They are the parents of two daughters and a son. Lorraine enjoys her special time with her grandchildren, as well as, reading, writing, painting, and traveling with her husband.

## Carol Carson

Carol A. Carson resides in North Carolina, has 2 children, 3 grandchildren, and 3 dogs. She is a Respiratory Therapist with a BS in Education. She is currently working for Duke University Health System in the Pulmonary Rehabilitation Department.

## Crystal Akins

Crystal Akins is the daughter of Claude Duell and of (the late) Bert Duell. She is one of two siblings who both have Cystic Fibrosis. She also is a wife and mother of one son. She resides in New York where she is a homemaker and enjoys life.

## Edwina Stratmon

Edwina Stratmon is married and has a twenty-three year old daughter. She received a dual lung transplant in 2004 at Duke University Medical Center. She and her family reside in Durham, North Carolina.

## Paula Thrush

Paula Thrush lives in Charleston, South Carolina, where her father, Lester Eckert, and her sister, Julie Thrush, also reside. She is the mother of two 11-year old male fat and sassy orange tabby cats, Timmay and CheezeBurger. Paula received a bilateral lung transplant on July 15, 2010, and is thrilled to finally have the ability, the energy and simply the breath to do the things she only dreamed of for so long.

## Kristina Kelso

Kristina Kelso of Boca Raton, FL. is the daughter of Fred and Mary Lou Bollin and sister of Frederick Bollin. Kristina has been married to Paul Kelso for 20 years and they have 2 wonderful kids, Jake 16 and Tatum 13. She enjoys spending time with her family and loving the new LIFE she's been given!

## Mary McCain

Mary Crisp McCain is married, has two grown children and two grandchildren. She received her lung transplant in November 2002 after years of dealing with the chronic disease Sarcoidosis. Mary attributes her survival to the many prayers by her family, friends and gifted physicians.

## Harry F. Collins, Jr.

Harry Collins is the son of Harry F. Collins Sr. and Dorothy H. Collins. He is one of two siblings and is the father of 1 daughter and 3 sons and the grandfather of 2 granddaughters, soon to be 5 grandchildren. He lives in Virginia where he works for JDSU and spends his spare time advocating for the Lung Transplant Foundation and raising money for research on rejection.

## Robert L. Shanks

Robert has been happily married to Ashley for 40 years. They have been blessed with two sons who are married, and they have

3 grandchildren. Robert's transplant was on Feb 4, 2010 and he and Ashley consider each day a gift full of exercise, cooking together, and serving those that God puts in their path. They live in Augusta, GA and vacation at Hilton Head, S.C. playing golf, riding bicycles, and walking on the beach.

## Melinda Anderson

Melinda Anderson, 48 years old, is a retired nurse since 1992. She has Cystic Fibrosis and received a double lung transplant and new lease on life on May 22, 2011. She lives in Lighthouse Point, FL with her boyfriend, Steve. Her interests are coaching women to follow their dreams and how to relate more deeply with people, volunteering, gardening, travelling and entertaining. One of her missions is to educate patients and caregivers on the benefits of aggressive-style chest physiotherapy as the gold standard of airway clearance and longevity.

## Perita Price

Perita Bryant Price is a former housing consultant, specializing in securing large dollar grants for large urban housing authorities through the US Dept. of Housing and Urban Development. Since being diagnosed with a chronic lung disease she has spent her time reading, writing, meditating and inspiring others to live their best life each and every day. Perita has two adult children, Bryant Anthony Price and Kristen Rose Price, and a grandson Elijah Anthony Umstead. She lives in Durham, NC.

## Brenda McDonald

Brenda McDonald lives each and every day to the fullest in Wilmington, NC and has a social media management and marketing company she began after the death of Ed while trying to find her way without him.

# Glossary

**A.R.D.S.**—*adult respiratory distress syndrome* ARDS usually occurs in people who are very ill with another disease or who have major injuries. Most people are already in the hospital when they develop ARDS.

**Abdominal aneurysm**—is a localized dilatation of the abdominal aorta exceeding the normal diameter by more than 50 percent, and is the most common form of aortic aneurysm

**Aftercare team**—those who care for a patient after a stay in the hospital

**Airlift(ed)**—is the organized delivery of supplies or personnel primarily via aircraft

**Airway constriction**—*bronchoconstriction* is the constriction of the airways in the lungs due to the tightening of surrounding smooth muscle, with consequent coughing, wheezing, and shortness of breath

**Allergist**—A medical practitioner specializing in the diagnosis and treatment of allergies

**Allergy and immunology doctor**—*see allergist*

**Anesthesia**—the condition of having sensation including pain blocked or temporarily taken away

**Anesthesiologist**—is a physician trained in anesthesia and peri-operative medicine

**Antibiotics**—A medicine (such as penicillin or its derivatives) that inhibits the growth of or destroys microorganisms

**Anvil, hammer and stirrup or stapes**—are the three smallest bones in the human body. They are contained within the middle ear space and serve to transmit sounds from the air to the fluid-filled labyrinth (cochlea)

**Asthma**—is the common chronic inflammatory disease of the airways characterized by variable and recurring symptoms, reversible airflow obstruction, and bronchospasm

**Attending Physician**—is a physician who has completed residency and practices medicine in a clinic or hospital, in the specialty learned during residency

**Atypical**—Not conforming to the normal type; Unusual or irregular

**B.I.D.**—means twice (two times) a day

**Biopsy**—is a medical test involving the removal of cells or tissues to be examined

**Bipap**—bi-level positive airway pressure) provides two levels of pressure: inspiratory positive airway pressure (IPAP) and a lower expiratory positive airway pressure (EPAP) for easier exhalation

**Bleb**—an irregular bulge in the plasma membrane of a cell

**Blood oxygen**—*see blood saturation*

**Blood oxygen saturation**—oxygen saturation refers to *oxygenation*, or when oxygen molecules (O2) enter the tissues of the body

**Blood pressure**—is the pressure exerted by circulating blood upon the walls of blood vessels, and is one of the principal vital signs

**Blood tests**—a laboratory analysis performed on a blood sample that is usually extracted from a vein in the arm using a needle, or via finger prick

**Blood work**—A medical process also known as a blood test

**Bloodletting**—is the withdrawal of often considerable quantities of blood from a patient to cure or prevent illness and disease. Bloodletting was based on an ancient system of medicine

**Breathing machine**—*see ventilator*

**Breathing treatments**—*see nebulizer*

**Bronchiectasis**—is a condition in which damage to the airways causes them to widen and become flabby and scarred.

**Bronchitis**—inflammation of the mucous membranes of the bronchi, the airways that carry airflow from the trachea into the lungs

**Bronchodilators**—a substance that dilates the bronchi and bronchioles, decreasing resistance in the respiratory airway and increasing airflow to the lungs

**Bronchoscope**—An instrument (bronchoscope) is inserted into the airways, usually through the nose or mouth, or occasionally through a tracheostomy

**Bronchoscopy**—a technique of visualizing the inside of the airways for diagnostic and therapeutic purposes

**Bronchus**—a passage of airway in the respiratory tract that conducts air into the lungs. The bronchus branches into smaller tubes, which in turn become bronchioles

**Cancer**—*see lung cancer*

**Carbon dioxide**—a naturally occurring chemical compound composed of two oxygen atoms covalently bonded to a single carbon atom

**Cardiac catherization**—is the insertion of a catheter into a chamber or vessel of the heart

**Cardiopulmonary**—of or relating to the heart and the lungs

**Cardiothoracic**—pertaining to organs inside the thorax (the chest)—generally treatment of conditions of the heart (heart disease) and lungs (lung disease)

**Cardiovascular exercise**—is physical exercise of relatively low intensity and long duration, which depends primarily on the aerobic energy system

**CAT scan**—special x-ray equipment with sophisticated computers to produce multiple images or pictures of the inside of the body

**Catherization**—(*heart cath*) is the insertion of a catheter into a chamber or vessel of the heart

**Catheters**—is a tube that can be inserted into a body cavity, duct, or vessel

**CF**—Cystic Fibrosis is an inherited disease of the secretory (see-KREH-tor-ee) glands. Secretory glands include glands that make mucus and sweat. CF mainly affects the lungs, pancreas, liver, intestines, sinuses, and sex organs

**Chest tubes**—a flexible plastic tube that is inserted through the side of the chest into the pleural space. It is used to remove air (pneumothorax) or fluid (pleural effusion, blood, chyle), or pus (empyema) from the intrathoracic space

**Chest x-rays**—a projection radiograph of the chest used to diagnose conditions affecting the chest, its contents, and nearby structures

**Chief of thoracic surgery**—*see thoracic surgery*

**Chief surgeon**—a surgeon appointed or elected head of the surgeons on the staff of a health care facility

**Chronic bronchitis**—a chronic inflammation of the bronchi (medium-size airways) in the lungs

**Chronic illness**—is an illness that is long-lasting or recurrent. It is usually applied to a condition that lasts more than three months

**Chronic lung disease**—*see chronic illness*

**CO2**—Carbon dioxide (chemical formula $CO_2$) is a naturally occurring chemical compound composed of two oxygen atoms covalently bonded to a single carbon atom

**Cognitive fog**—unusually poor mental function, associated with confusion, forgetfulness and difficulty concentrating

**Congestive heart failure**—the inability of the heart to supply sufficient blood flow to meet the needs of the body

**COPD**—*Chronic Obstructive Pulmonary* is a progressive disease that makes it hard to breathe. COPD can cause coughing that produces large amounts of mucus, wheezing, shortness of breath, chest tightness, and other symptoms

**Critical Care nursing**—the field of nursing with a focus on the utmost care of the critically ill or unstable patients

**CT scan**—*see CAT scan*

**Cuffed trach**—*see tracheotomy*

**Cuffed-less trach**—*see tracheotomy*

**Cultures**—the propagation of microorganisms or of living tissue cells in special media conducive to their growth

**Cyanosis**—is the appearance of a blue or purple coloration of the skin or mucous membranes due to the tissues near the skin surface being low on oxygen

**Cystic Fibrosis**—*see CF*

**Dermatologist**—one who takes care of diseases, in the widest sense, and some cosmetic problems of the skin, scalp, hair, and nails

**Deviated septum**—a common physical disorder of the nose, involving a displacement of the nasal septum

**Diabetes**—is a group of metabolic diseases in which a person has high blood sugar, either because the body does not produce enough insulin, or because cells do not respond to the insulin that is produced

**Diabetic**—*see Diabetes*

**Digestive tract**—refers to the stomach and intestine, and sometimes to all the structures from the mouth to the anus

**Double lung transplant**—*see lung transplant*

**Drainage tubes**—*see chest tubes*

**Dry-run**—is a testing process where the effects of a possible failure are intentionally mitigated

**Echocardiogram**—is a sonogram of the heart

**ED**—*see Emergency Room*

**Emergency room**—*see ED*

**Emphysema**—a long-term, progressive disease of the lungs that primarily causes shortness of breath. In people with emphysema, the tissues necessary to support the physical shape and function of the lungs are destroyed

**ENT doctor**—Otolaryngology or ENT (ear, nose and throat) is the branch of medicine that specializes in the diagnosis and treatment of ear, nose, throat, and head and neck disorders

**ENT surgeon**—*see ENT doctor*

**Esophagus**—The muscular membranous tube for the passage of food from the pharynx to the stomach

**Exacerbations**—A worsening. In medicine, exacerbation may refer to an increase in the severity of a disease or its signs and symptoms

**Feeding tube**—is a medical device used to provide nutrition to patients who cannot obtain nutrition by swallowing

**Femoral aneurysm**—is bulging and weakness in the wall of the femoral artery, located in the thigh. A femoral aneurysm can burst, which may cause life-threatening uncontrolled bleeding.

**Fibrosis**—is the formation of excess fibrous connective tissue in an organ or tissue in a reparative or reactive process

**Flolan®**—is a sterile sodium salt formulated for intravenous (IV) administration

**Full liquid diet**—A full or strained liquid diet consists of both clear and opaque liquid foods with a smooth consistency

**Fungus**—is a member of a large group of eukaryotic organisms that includes microorganisms such as yeasts and molds

**Googled**—**to google** (also spelled **to Google**) refers to using the Google search engine to obtain information on the Web

**Granuloma**—is a medical term for a roughly spherical mass of immune cells that forms when the immune system attempts to wall off substances that it perceives as foreign but is unable to eliminate

**Hand-held inhalers**—A metered dose inhaler, usually called an inhaler, is a canister of medication that is under pressure. The canister is attached to a mouthpiece. The inhaler releases a mist of medication in a preset dose

**Heart catheterization**—is the insertion of a catheter into a chamber or vessel of the heart. This is done for both investigational and interventional purposes

**Heart scan**—provides pictures of your heart's arteries (coronary arteries)

**Hickman catheter**—is an intravenous catheter most often used for the administration of chemotherapy or other medications, as well as for the withdrawal of blood for analysis. Hickman lines may remain in place for extended periods and are used when long-term intravenous access is needed

**High resolution chest CAT scan**—or *HRCT* of the lung is a medical diagnostic test used for diagnosis and assessment of interstitial lung disease

**Hyperventilating**—*see hyperventilation*

**Hyperventilation**—or *overbreathing* is the state of increased respiratory rate in a person

IBM®—is an American multinational technology and consulting firm headquartered in Armonk, New York. IBM manufactures and sells computer hardware and software, and it offers infrastructure, hosting and consulting services in areas ranging from mainframe computers to nanotechnology.[2]

ICU—is a specialized department in a hospital that provides intensive-care medicine

Idiopathic Pulmonary Fibrosis (cause unknown)—is a chronic, progressive form of lung disease characterized by fibrosis of the supporting framework (interstitium) of the lungs

Immunosuppressive therapy—Immunosuppression involves an act that reduces the activation or efficacy of the immune system

Immunotherapy—is a medical term defined as the treatment of disease by inducing, enhancing, or suppressing an immune response

Infectious Disease doctor—a doctor of internal medicine (or, in some cases, pediatrics) who is qualified as an expert in the diagnosis and treatment of infectious diseases

Inhaler—*see hand held inhaler*

Insulin—is a hormone central to regulating carbohydrate and fat metabolism in the body

Intensive Care unit—*see ICU*

Internist—Physicians specializing in internal medicine are called *internists*

Interns—a recent medical graduate receiving supervised training in a hospital as an assistant physician

**Interstitial Lung Disease**—also known as *diffuse parenchymal lung disease (DPLD)*,[1] refers to a group of lung diseases affecting the interstitium (the tissue and space around the air sacs of the lungs)

**Intubation**—is the insertion of a tube into an external or internal orifice of the body for the purpose of adding or removing fluids or air

**IV**—is the giving of substances directly into a vein. The word intravenous simply means "within a vein"

**IV antibiotics**—Intravenous antibiotics are antibiotic medications designed to be delivered directly into the bloodstream

**IV catheter**—*see catheter*

**Job**—The Book of Job commonly referred to simply as *Job*, is one of the books of the Hebrew Bible

**Kidney stones**—are solid concretions or crystal aggregations formed in the kidneys from dietary minerals in the urine

**Life support**—in medicine is a broad term that applies to any therapy used to sustain a patient's life while they are critically ill or injured

**Lip biopsy**—*see biopsy*

**Liver biopsy**—*see biopsy*

**Lobe**—a clear anatomical division or extension that can be determined without the use of a microscope (at the gross anatomy level)

**Lobectomy**—means *surgical excision of a lobe*. This may refer to a lobe of the lung, a lobe of the thyroid (hemithyroidectomy), or a lobe of the brain (as in anterior temporal lobectomy)

**Lung cancer**—is a disease that consists of uncontrolled cell growth in tissues of the lung

**Lung capacity**—refer to the volume of air associated with different phases of the respiratory cycle. Lung volumes are directly measured. Lung capacities are inferred from lung volumes

**Lung function**—(or *pulmonary function test (PFT)* is a test to measure the function of the lungs

**Lung scan**—is a nuclear scanning test that is most commonly used to detect a blood clot that is preventing normal blood flow to part of a lung

**Lung transplant**—is a surgical procedure in which a patient's diseased lungs are partially or totally replaced by lungs which come from a donor

**Lung Transplant Foundation (LTF).**—The non-profit organization focused on advancing Lung Transplant research. https://lungtransplantfoundation.org

**Lymph nodes**—is a small ball or an oval-shaped organ of the immune system, distributed widely throughout the body including the armpit and stomach/gut and linked by lymphatic vessels

**Lyrica®—Pregabalin** (INN) (pronounced /pri'gæbəlin/) is an anticonvulsant drug used for neuropathic pain and as an adjunct therapy for partial seizures with or without secondary generalization in adults.[1] It has also been found effective for generalized anxiety disorder and is (as of 2007) approved for this use in the European Union.[1] It was designed as a more potent successor to gabapentin. Pregabalin is marketed by Pfizer under the trade name **Lyrica**

**Mastoid bone**—The mastoid bone is a bone located behind the ear (felt as a hard bump behind the ear). Inside it looks like a honeycomb, with the spaces filled with air.

**Mastoidectomy**—A mastoidectomy is a surgical procedure designed to remove infection or growths in the bone behind the ear (mastoid bone). Its purpose is to create a "safe" ear and prevent further damage to the hearing apparatus.

**Medical record**—a systematic documentation of a single patient's long-term individual medical history and care

**Methotrexate®**—abbreviated **MTX** and formerly known as **amethopterin**, is an antimetabolite and antifolate drug. It is used in treatment of cancer, autoimmune diseases, ectopic pregnancy, and for the induction of medical abortions.

**Morphine drip**—morphine administered to a patient by machine for comfort measures

**Moses, David, and Lot**—the names of people mentioned in The Holy Bible

**MRI**—is a medical imaging technique used in radiology to visualize detailed internal structures

**MRSA**—is a strain of *Staphylococcus aureus* (*S. aureus*) bacteria. *S. aureus* is a common type of bacteria that normally live on the skin and sometimes in the nasal passages of healthy people

**Muscle relaxers**—is a drug which affects skeletal muscle function and decreases the muscle tone. It may be used to alleviate symptoms such as muscle spasms, pain, and hyperreflexia.

**Nasal cannula**—is a device used to deliver supplemental oxygen or airflow to a patient or person in need of respiratory help. This device consists of a plastic tube which fits behind the ears, and a set of two prongs which are placed in the nostrils

**National Transplant List**—is the private, non-profit organization that manages the nation's organ transplant system under contract with the federal government

**Nebulizer**—is a device used to administer medication in the form of a mist inhaled into the lungs

**Nebulizer treatments**—are called breathing/ aerosol treatments or med nebs. Allows medicine to go more deeply into your airways because of the fine particle size. The treatments help you breathe easier using medicines called bronchodilators that open the airway passages

**Neurology neurologist**—is a medical specialty dealing with disorders of the nervous system

**Nodule**—refers to a relatively hard, roughly spherical abnormal structure.

**Non-Specific Interstitial Pneumonia (NSIP)**—is a form of idiopathic interstitial pneumonia.

**O2**—*the symbol for Oxygen . . . see oxygen*

**Occluded**—closed off; "an occluded artery

**Organ donation**—the donation of biological tissue or an organ of the human body, from a living or dead person to a living recipient in need of a transplantation

**Oxycontin®**—an opioid analgesic medication synthesized from opium-derived thebaine. Generally prescribed for relief from moderate to severe pain

**Oxygen**—At standard temperature and pressure, two atoms of the element bind to form dioxygen, a very pale blue, odorless, tasteless diatomic gas with the formula O2. Oxygen is essential for cell metabolism, and in turn, tissue oxygenation is essential for all normal physiological functions.[1]

**Oxygen Saturation**—is a relative measure of the amount of oxygen that is dissolved or carried in a given medium

**Oxygen therapy**—is the administration of oxygen as a medical intervention, which can be for a variety of purposes in both chronic and acute patient

**PA**—*see physician assistant*

**Pathology report**—is a written medical document which describes the analysis of specimens by the pathologist.

**Pet scan**—is a nuclear medicine imaging technique that produces a three-dimensional image or picture of functional processes in the body

**PH (*Pulmonary Hypertension*)**—is an increase in blood pressure in the pulmonary artery, pulmonary vein, or pulmonary capillaries, together known as the lung vasculature, leading to shortness of breath, dizziness, fainting, and other symptoms, all of which are exacerbated by exertion.

**Phlegm**—is a liquid secreted by the mucous membranes of mammalians. Its definition is limited to the mucus produced by the respiratory system, excluding that from the nasal passages, and particularly that which is expelled by coughing(sputum)

**Physical therapists**—*see physical therapy*

**Physical therapy**—is a health care profession which aims the physical treatment and management of disease or condition which enables people to reach their maximum potential

**PA (*Physician Assistant*)**—is a healthcare professional trained and licensed to practice medicine with limited supervision of a physician

**Picturesque**—Visually attractive, esp. in a quaint or pretty style

**Pleural space**—the *pleural cavity* is the body cavity that surrounds the lungs. The thin space between the two pleural layers is known as the pleural cavity

**Pneumonia**—Lung inflammation caused by bacterial or viral infection

**Portable oxygen**—a system that provides you with the freedom to leave your home and move about untethered. Its oxygen may be compressed or liquid

**Post-surgical infections**—infections that one contracts after a surgical procedure

**Post-transplant coordinator**—will work with the surgeon to oversee your medical care during your hospital stay following transplant.

**Prednisone**—is a synthetic corticosteroid drug that is particularly effective as an immunosuppressant drug. It is used to treat certain inflammatory diseases and (at higher doses) some types of cancer, but has significant adverse effects. Because it suppresses the immune system, it leaves patients more susceptible to infections

**Primary care provider**—or PCP, is a physician/medical doctor who provides both the first contact for a person with an undiagnosed health concern as well as continuing care of varied medical conditions

**Prognosis**—is a medical term to describe the likely outcome of an illness.

**Prograf®**—is an immunosuppressive drug that is mainly used after allogeneic organ transplant to reduce the activity of the patient's immune system and so lower the risk of organ rejection

**Protonix®**—is a proton pump inhibitor drug used for short-term treatment of erosion and ulceration of the esophagus caused by gastroesophageal reflux disease

**Pseudomonas**—A bacterium of a genus that occurs in soil and detritus (detritus generally refers to any disintegrated material or debris. Within the field of biology), including a number that are pathogens of plants or animals

**Pulmonary artery**—carry deoxygenated blood from the heart to the lungs. They are the only arteries (other than umbilical arteries in the fetus) that carry deoxygenated blood

**Pulmonary disease**—*see lung disease*

**Pulmonary embolism**—(*PE*) is a blockage of the main artery of the lung or one of its branches by a substance that has travelled from elsewhere in the body through the bloodstream (embolism)

**Pulmonary function numbers**—*see pulmonary function tests*

**pulmonary function test**—are a group of tests that measure how well the lungs take in and release air and how well they move gases such as oxygen from the atmosphere into the body's circulation

**Pulmonary Hypertension**—*see PH*

**Pulmonary rehabilitation graduate program**—a program for patients who have completed any of other three programs offered at the Duke Center for Living

**Pulmonary rehabilitation**—is an integral part of the clinical management and health maintenance of those patients with chronic respiratory disease who remain symptomatic or continue to have decreased function despite standard medical treatment

**Pulmonologist**—is the specialty that deals with diseases of the respiratory tract and respiratory disease

**Pulseoximeter**—is a medical device that indirectly monitors the oxygen saturation of a patient's blood. It is often attached to a medical monitor so staff can see a patient's oxygenation at all times

**RAT-G treatment**—type of chemo that attaches to the t-cells to stop the rejection in organ transplant patients
**Real lung biopsy**—removes a small piece of lung tissue which can be looked at under a microscope

**Reflux disease, or G.E.R.D**—is chronic symptoms or mucosal damage caused by stomach acid coming up from the stomach into the esophagus

**Reproductive system**—is a system of organs within an organism which work together for the purpose of reproduction.

**Respiratory system**—is the anatomical system of an organism that introduces respiratory gases to the interior and performs gas exchange

**Respiratory therapy**—is an allied health field involved in the assessment and treatment of breathing disorders including chronic lung problems

**RSV**—is a virus that causes respiratory tract infections

**Sarcoid growth/granulomas**—a sarcoma like tumor; fleshlike

**Sarcoidosis**—is a disease in which abnormal collections of chronic inflammatory cells (granulomas) form as nodules in multiple organs.

**Saturation levels**—*SEE OXYGEN SATURATION*

**Scar tissue**—a product of healing in major wounds

**Sculpturesque**—resembling sculpture

**Serratia infection**—refers to a disease caused by a species in the genus Serratia, rod-shaped bacteria of the Enterobacteriaceae family

**Sleep Apnea**—is a sleep disorder characterized by abnormal pauses in breathing or instances of abnormally low breathing, during sleep

**Sleep study test**—are tests that watch what happens to your body during sleep. The studies are done to find out what is causing your sleep problems

**Solumedrol**—used to treat certain conditions associated with decreased adrenal gland function. It is also used to treat severe inflammation caused by certain conditions. It works by modifying the body's immune response to various conditions and decreasing inflammation

**Speech therapy**—treatment for speech and/or language disorders

**Spontaneous pneumothorax**—when a lung collapses without any cause. A small area in the lung that is filled with air, called a bleb, ruptures, and the air leaks into the space around the lung

**Staphylococcus**—tend to grow in grapelike clusters, they are constantly present on the skin or in the upper respiratory tract and are the most common cause of localized suppurating infections

**Stent**—a mold for keeping a skin graph in place. A tubular support placed temporarily inside a blood vessel, canal, or duct to aid healing or relieve an obstruction

**Step down of prednisone**—prednisone taper is a decrease in your dose by a tiny amount, usually half a pill or 2.5mg. This is due to the fact that being on a corticosteroid like prednisone suppresses the adrenal glands

**Steroidal injections**—involves the injecting of corticosteroid (steroids for short) into one or two specific areas of inflammation allows the doctor to deliver a high dose of medication directly to the bothersome area

**Nissan fundoplication**—*also known as stomach wrap* . . . the upper curve of the stomach (the fundus) is wrapped around the esophagus and sewn into place so that the lower portion of the esophagus passes through a small tunnel of stomach muscle. This surgery strengthens the valve between the esophagus and stomach (lower esophageal sphincter), which stops acid from backing up into the esophagus as easily. This allows the esophagus to heal

**Stress fracture**—is one type of incomplete fracture in bones. It is caused by "unusual or repeated stress" and also heavy continuous weight on the ankle or leg

**Suction**—The drawing of a fluid or solid into a space because the pressure inside of it is lower than that outside.

**Suctioning**—removal of material through the use of negative pressure as in suctioning an operative wound during and after surgery to remove exudates or suctioning of the respiratory passages to remove secretions that the patient cannot remove by coughing

**Supplemental oxygen**—*see oxygen therapy*

**Surgical intensive care unit**—provide holistic care to critically ill patients. It is a 10-bed adult critical care unit designed to provide comprehensive care for critically ill surgical and trauma patients

**Swallow test**—Tests your doctor or specialist use to determine the cause of a swallowing problem. They may use a **Barium**

**X-ray, Endoscopy.** fiber-optic endoscopic evaluation of swallowing (FEES), or **Esophageal muscle test.**

**Thoracic aortic aneurysm**—When a weak area of your thoracic aorta expands or bulges, it is called a thoracic aortic aneurysm (TAA). They can rupture or burst and cause severe internal bleeding that can lead to shock or death

**Thoracic hemorrhage**—*see thoracic aneurysm*

**Thoracic surgery**—The field of medicine involved in the surgical treatment of diseases affecting organs inside the thorax (the chest). Generally treatment of conditions of the lungs, chest wall, and diaphragm.

**Toupet procedure**—is a surgical procedure to treat gastroesophageal reflux disease (GERD) and hiatus hernia.

**Trach**—*see trachea*

**Trachea**—is a tube that connects the pharynx or larynx to the lungs, allowing the passage of air

**Tracheostomy**—surgical procedure to create an opening through the neck into the trachea (windpipe). A tube is usually placed through this opening to provide an airway and to remove secretions from the lungs

**Tracheotomy**—consists of making an incision on the anterior aspect of the neck and opening a direct airway through an incision in the trachea. The resulting stoma can serve independently as an airway or as a site for a tracheostomy tube to be inserted; this tube allows a person to breathe without the use of his or her nose or mouth

**Transplant Coordinator**—oversees the organ transplant process. This includes locating donor organs; arranging transportation for organs; coordinating transplants; consulting with physicians, surgeons, and hospital staff; and conferring with and counseling recipients and recipients' families

**Trial study**—are test or experiment. An experiment performed on human beings in order to evaluate the comparative efficacy of two or more therapies

**Trigeminal nerve**—is responsible for sensation in the face. Sensory information from the face and body is processed by parallel pathways in the central nervous system. It is the fifth cranial nerve

**Trigeminal neuralgia**—is a neuropathic disorder characterized by episodes of intense pain in the face, originating from the trigeminal nerve

**True lung biopsy**—*see lung biopsy*

**Typical IPF**—Having the distinctive qualities of a particular type of person or thing. A chronic, progressive form of lung disease characterized by fibrosis of the supporting framework (interstitium) of the lungs. By definition, the term is used only when the cause of the pulmonary fibrosis is unknown ("idiopathic")

**Ultrasound**—is cyclic sound pressure with a frequency greater than the upper limit of human hearing, used in medicine in the technique of Ultrasonography

**United Network for Organ Sharing**—is a non-profit, scientific and educational organization that administers the only Organ Procurement and Transplantation Network (OPTN) in the United States, established (42 U.S.C. § 274) by the U.S. Congress in 1984.

**Valium ®**—mainly used to treat anxiety, insomnia, and symptoms of acute alcohol withdrawal. It is also used as a premedication for inducing sedation, anxiolysis or amnesia before certain medical procedures. Trademark for a preparation of diazepam, an anxiolytic and skeletal muscle relaxant

**Ventilator**—an apparatus designed to mechanically move breathable air into and out of the lungs, to provide the mechanism of breathing for a patient who is physically unable to breathe, or breathing insufficiently

**Virus**—is a small infectious agent that can replicate only inside the living cells of organisms

**VQ scan**—A *ventilation/perfusion lung scan*, is a type of medical imaging using scintigraphy and medical isotopes to evaluate the circulation of air and blood within a patient's lungs, in order to determine the ventilation/perfusion ratio

**XOLAIR®**—XOLAIR® (omalizumab) for subcutaneous use is an injectable, prescription medicine for patients 12 years of age and older. It is for patients with moderate to severe persistent allergic asthma caused by year-round allergens in the air. XOLAIR is for patients who are not controlled by asthma medicines called inhaled steroids

http://www.nhlbi.nih.gov
http://en.wikipedia.org/wiki
Mosby's Medical Dictionary, 8th edition. © 2009, Elsevier.
http://www.acponline.org/patients_families/about_internal_medicine/subspecialties/infectious_disease/
http://www.ask.com/questions-about/Intravenous-Antibiotics
http://www.webmd.com/lung/lung-scan
http://www.pediatric-ent.com/learning/surgeries/mastoidectomy.htm
Based on WordNet 3.0, Farlex clipart collection. © 2003-2008 Princeton University, Farlex Inc.
http://nyp.org/health/pathology-report.html
http://emedicine.medscape.com/article/319885-overview

.

Printed in the United States
by Baker & Taylor Publisher Services